When Your Child Has Lyme Disease
A Parent's Survival Guide

*Practical strategies for coping with an illness
that can be shattering to family life*

By
Sandra K. Berenbaum, LCSW, BCD, and
Dorothy Kupcha Leland

Lyme Literate Press
Davis, California

When Your Child Has Lyme Disease
A Parent's Survival Guide

Published by Lyme Literate Press
www.lymeliteratepress.com

ISBN 978-0-9962243-0-7 (paperback)
ISBN 978-0-9962243-1-4 (e-book)

Library of Congress Control Number: 2015937451

Dedications

Sandy:

To my grandmother, Devorah Bannett, of blessed memory
who taught me how to love,
And to my husband, Lenny, my children and grandchildren,
who I love with all my heart

Dorothy:

To Bob, Jeremy, and Rachel, who brighten my days

Authors' Note

When Your Child Has Lyme Disease: A Parent's Survival Guide is based on the personal and professional experiences of the authors in coping with Lyme disease. One of the authors, Sandra K. Berenbaum, LCSW, BCD, is a psychotherapist whose practice focuses on Lyme disease and other tick-borne illnesses, and the other author, Dorothy Kupcha Leland, is a Lyme disease activist. Both have experienced the challenges of Lyme disease personally or through the illness of their loved ones.

The authors share the practical strategies that they have developed and used in their own lives and, in the case of Sandra Berenbaum, in her professional practice as well. However, this book is not intended as a substitute for medical and mental health advice and treatment, and the strategies may not be appropriate for every reader. For that reason, this book does not and cannot take the place of consultation with or treatment by an appropriate healthcare professional. Readers are urged to seek professional advice before making use of any of the contents of this book to make sure that it is appropriate for them.

All names and various other identifying details about individuals who are mentioned in examples drawn from Sandra Berenbaum's professional practice have been changed. In some instances, the examples are composites of several individuals. For that reason, any resemblance between such individuals and real persons is strictly coincidental. Dorothy Leland has used the real names of her adult children, Rachel and Jeremy, with their permission. Three treating doctors who kindly spoke with the authors are identified in the text with pseudonyms. Otherwise, whenever a book, lecture or website is cited as a source, only real names are used.

Contents

Foreword by Dr. Richard Horowitz

WE ARE IN THE MIDDLE of a spreading epidemic of tick-borne diseases in the United States, creating a health care crisis affecting millions of people. I am a board-certified internist who has seen over 12,000 cases of Lyme disease in the past 28 years. I have witnessed firsthand the tremendous suffering that families go through with this illness, either getting a proper diagnosis and/or finding an effective treatment. Lyme disease, as most chronic illnesses, can create difficulties as well as opportunities for growth and healing if we know how to skillfully work with the experiences presented to us. Unfortunately, most of us have not been trained to deal with the issues that Lyme disease brings.

Children with Lyme present specific challenges. There are physical, emotional, and mental burdens that children and families must deal with as they navigate the maze of pursuing proper medical care. Children may have physical symptoms, such as fatigue, headaches, joint and muscle pains, preventing them from going to school. They may suffer from insomnia and cognitive difficulties that may be quite extreme. Many experience depression and anxiety caused by the illness itself, as well as from the emotional burden of not going to school and being with friends. The inability to have a normal childhood and live up to self-expectations and/or the expectations of others can be a daunting experience for both children and parents. Skillful emotional support and guidance, as well as an understanding of how to meet educational needs and manage day-to-day family life, is essential in Lyme. We need a structured and comprehensive support system in place for families to navigate the difficult waters of Lyme and chronic illness. We finally have that guidance in this book.

The authors have worked in this field for many years, and their combined knowledge and wisdom are now available to help families

1

like yours grow through the experience. This is not a medical book, but is instead a roadmap for mothers and fathers, giving you practical strategies for parenting a child with Lyme, as well as how to cope yourself with the challenges of day-to-day family life.

The co-authors share their knowledge from different perspectives. Sandy Berenbaum is a psychotherapist who has worked intimately with families coping with Lyme disease for over 20 years. After witnessing those struggles firsthand, she has developed a unique protocol for helping others, called "responsive psychotherapy." On the other hand, Dorothy Leland represents the parent's point of view. She has negotiated the challenges of Lyme in her own family for over a decade, while moderating a Lyme support group, and writing a popular blog called *Touched by Lyme*. This book contains the insights of their combined decades of experience. It is designed to help support you with one of the most challenging experiences of your family life. Please read it carefully, mixing its wisdom with self-compassion as you are guided on your family's journey towards healing and wholeness.

—*Dr. Richard Horowitz, August 2, 2015*

Preface: Why We Wrote This Book

Dorothy Leland:

In 2005, out of the blue, my then-13-year-old daughter became so disabled from a mysterious condition that she was forced to use a wheelchair. At that time, I didn't even know what Lyme disease was. I didn't know that our family had fallen into a huge medical controversy, what many have dubbed "The Lyme Wars." I didn't know we'd have to battle a medical system that denied her illness. And I did not anticipate the many complex personal and family issues that would arise. We felt alone. But, in fact, we were part of a growing yet invisible group—families grappling with a disease that is ignored by our government and the medical establishment.

It was a long, hard, expensive slog but, eventually, we got through it. We were guided by Internet research and online patient support groups. In time, we found our way to medical practitioners and treatments that put our daughter's health back on track and allowed her to leave that wheelchair behind for good. At that point, I entered the world of Lyme disease activism. I founded a patient support group, started a blog called *Touched by Lyme*, and now advocate for the rights of Lyme patients with the national organization LymeDisease.org.

Through these activities, I regularly encounter parents who face the same issues my family did. Many of them are in even more daunting circumstances. The purpose of this book is to shorten the learning curve for parents and family members of children with Lyme disease. I hope it will help them find a path to healing for everyone in the family.

Sandy Berenbaum:

In 1984, I was a psychotherapist in private practice, working with adolescents and their families. I began to experience severe migraine headaches, which worsened over the next six years. None of the specialists I consulted could help me. Then, one day in 1990, I could not hold water in my mouth when I brushed my teeth, because the right side of my face was paralyzed. This was Bell's palsy, a common symptom of Lyme disease. I started treatment with one the few Lyme specialists in the country at that time. As it turned out, migraines and a paralyzed face were not my only Lyme-related problems. I also had trouble with sleep, fatigue, concentration, and memory. It took four years of antibiotic therapy to resolve these symptoms.

As I learned more about how Lyme disease can affect the body and the brain, I began to wonder whether some of my young clients might also be infected. After all, since we lived in New York's highly Lyme-endemic Hudson Valley, we were all exposed to ticks. To my surprise, many of my clients indeed had Lyme at the root of their physical and psychological problems.

As I worked with these adolescents and their parents, I saw the enormous toll Lyme disease takes on whole families. At that time, I knew of no other psychotherapy practices that focused on the unique challenges faced by families of children with Lyme disease. Nor could I find any medical journals that addressed these issues. Thus, my clients and I had to build the road as we traveled on it. Together with my clients, I developed what I now call "responsive psychotherapy," which is specifically geared towards helping families grappling with tick-borne illnesses.

This book is aimed at parents and other family members of children who are ill with tick-borne diseases. However, I hope mental health practitioners will read it, too. If so, I hope it inspires them to look closely at the possibility of a medical cause for a patient's "mental illness."

How our chapters are organized

At different spots throughout the book, we indicate whose voice is telling the story. We believe that maintaining our separate viewpoints—as health care professional and parent of a child with Lyme—strengthens our message. Parts of Dorothy Leland's sections have been previously published in her blog, *Touched by Lyme.*

one

Falling Down Alice's Rabbit Hole

Dorothy:

On March 12, 2005, my then-13-year-old daughter, Rachel, fell and sprained her wrist in a soccer game. It hurt too much for her to continue playing, so she sat on the sidelines with an ice pack and cheered her team to victory. None of us realized how drastically our lives would change from that moment onward. At that time, we thought she'd be back playing soccer after a few days of icing her wrist and taking ibuprofen.

The following week, Rachel started having severe pains in her knees, and we iced those too. And then one ankle hurt so much she couldn't put weight on her foot. X-rays showed nothing amiss, and we were advised to keep icing and giving ibuprofen. We finally rented a wheelchair, so she could get from one end of her junior high school campus to the other.

A few days later, Rachel called me from the school office in tears. "My foot feels like it's on fire!" she sobbed. A call to the doctor's office got us in for a battery of blood tests that day, and an appointment with a rheumatologist the next. He said it was juvenile rheumatoid arthritis and prescribed prednisone, which suppresses the immune system. He also ordered more tests, including a full body scan.

This was such a confusing, scary time for the whole family. Rachel's weird symptoms came and went capriciously. Sometimes one foot hurt, sometimes the other. Sometimes she felt electrical shocks in her elbow. Sometimes one foot felt as cold as ice to my touch, while the other one felt warm. What never varied was a searing pain in her wrist, knees, and ankles. It was difficult to reassure my frightened, suffering daughter when I was so frightened and suffering myself.

A neighbor asked if Rachel had ever been tested for Lyme disease. He knew someone with similar symptoms who was eventually diagnosed with Lyme. I went to my computer and typed "Lyme disease" into Google. Some information I found seemed to fit our situation, but most was contradictory and confusing. I made a mental note to ask the doctor about it.

In the meantime, we did the lab work and had the scan done. Following the doctor's instructions, we started her on prednisone. Almost immediately, things got dramatically worse. On her second day of that medication, Rachel collapsed on the floor and could barely move. I managed to get her onto the couch, called the rheumatologist's office and told the nurse I thought we should stop the prednisone. She said she'd talk to the doctor and get back to me. Almost as an afterthought, I said, "Can we have her tested for Lyme disease?"

The nurse soon called me back, offering an appointment the next day.

I said, "And what about a Lyme disease test?"

"The doctor says there's no need to test, because she doesn't have Lyme disease."

I hung up the phone, perplexed. How in the world could he possibly know that?

This was my first direct experience with what I came to call the "Alice-down-the-Lyme-rabbit-hole" phenomenon—the weird and dysfunctional way the medical establishment approaches Lyme disease. I didn't know then how big a part of our lives it would become.

The next day, the rheumatologist seemed annoyed that I'd stopped giving Rachel the prednisone. And he appeared chagrined to admit that the various tests results didn't indicate juvenile rheumatoid arthritis. He recommended switching from ibuprofen to naproxen (a different non-steroidal anti-inflammatory medication). Period. No further tests, no other treatments. He practically said, "Don't let the door hit you on the way out."

My child was a crumpled heap of pain and misery and that was all he had to offer? Not even a referral to a different specialist?

I cleared my throat and ventured tentatively, "I'd like to ask about Lyme disease."

His body visibly stiffened. "She doesn't have Lyme disease." It came out like a low growl. He turned away, as if to signal the end of the conversation.

Why was he acting so strangely? "Why do you say that? What do you base it on?"

He tersely replied: "There's no Lyme disease around here."

That's all? From my cursory research, I knew Lyme disease is spread by infected ticks, and that there were known cases in California.

"We don't spend all our time here," I stammered in surprise. "We hike, we camp. We've gone to different states, even out of the country."

"It doesn't matter. THERE'S NO LYME AROUND HERE!"

My daughter looked like she was going to cry. The doctor looked like he was going to pop a blood vessel. As we left, I felt like we'd somehow been transported to Bizarro World.

7

Despite the rheumatologist, my husband and I pushed to have Rachel tested for Lyme anyway. However, when the results came back negative, that ended any consideration of Lyme disease.

Spring turned to summer. We saw more doctors, who prescribed strong medications. The drugs made Rachel dizzy and nauseated, but did nothing to reduce the pain, now in her neck, back, knees, and ankles. She also developed an extreme hypersensitivity in her upper back and shoulders. Even a feather-light touch, she said, "felt like being stung by a thousand bees."

None of the doctors or medical tests could shed light on what was wrong. A prestigious children's hospital put her through an intensive physical therapy program after the hospital staff concluded her pain was "psychological." If she could grit her way through it, they insisted, the pain would subside. Mind over matter. The process yielded a modicum of success, since by the end of her month's stay, she could walk haltingly for short distances. The hospital staff took this as proof that they were on the right track, and I was thrilled to see my daughter on her feet again. But Rachel told me tearfully that everything hurt as much as ever. Later, she would refer to this as "the time of pretend walking."

Shortly before we left the hospital, her doctors called me into a private conference. They told me that my attitude was contributing heavily to Rachel's health problems. They said my misguided belief that something "real" was causing Rachel's pain prevented her from getting past it. They said I could best help her by recognizing that there was nothing physically wrong with her, and that she had developed a psychological need to be in a wheelchair. Enabling her in the use of that emotional crutch would be destructive. We mustn't "give in" or "coddle" her in any way. She should continue with twice-weekly physical therapy sessions at home, as well as psychological counseling. They

8

would transfer her care back to our local medical group, and further questions should be taken up with her doctor at home.

Their words hit like a sharp punch in the gut. *This was my fault?* Practically overnight, my daughter had gone from being healthy, happy, and athletic into being in a state of constant pain. My efforts to help her were actually hurting her? It didn't make sense. Rachel had been suffering—our whole family had been suffering along with her—for five long months. Five months of her pain and my dogged determination to leave no stone unturned in trying to fix it. Now, they said, my desire to help my daughter was making it worse?

Stunned, confused and wounded by their words, I tried not to burst into tears. Could I have done something differently? Was I not supposed to look for answers? They were right about one thing. I did believe something "real" was causing this. However, at that point, after two negative tests, I'd accepted that it wasn't Lyme disease. But now, they said my very search for answers was impeding her progress. I couldn't process what they were telling me. On the drive home, I tried not to think about it.

Back home, we followed the hospital's treatment protocol to the letter, at first. Per doctors' instructions, the wheelchair was banished. Twice a week, I carted Rachel to physical therapy. Twice a week, she saw her psychotherapist. When eighth grade started that fall, I drove her to school and dropped her off as close to her first class as possible. It was a huge ordeal for her to walk haltingly from one class to another. She'd arrive late for each class, exhausted, her increasing pain distracting her from learning math, English, or anything else. At PE time, she sat alone in the library.

Her pain increased. During one particular physical therapy session, she felt something pull in her lower back. From then on, she had a new symptom: it hurt too much to sit up straight in a chair or lie down flat in a bed. The only way she got any relief at all was to be at a slant, like in a reclining chair. The physical therapist examined her and said there was nothing wrong. An MRI of her back was "unremarkable," meaning it showed nothing amiss.

Because Rachel could no longer lie flat, it was practically impossible for her to sleep. We experimented by propping her up with pillows in different ways. Some configurations helped a bit. I asked the physical therapist (PT) about getting a hospital bed to allow Rachel to sleep with her back at a slant. The PT was horrified at my suggestion. No hospital bed! That would be "giving in" to her.

By now, even the most limited "pretend walking" was too much for Rachel. At home, we used a wheeled office chair to push her from bedroom to bathroom. We knew the doctors wouldn't approve, but it seemed prudent to save her energies for walking at school. Yet soon, school was simply too difficult. Eventually, all the pain, suffering, anger, and frustration boiled over into emotional outbursts, screaming fits directed mostly at her Dad and me. As I looked at my daughter's beautiful face distorted in agony, heard her animal-like howls that seemed to come from some place profoundly within her, I wanted to shriek too. But I tamped down my own fears—that Rachel might never get better, that our family might never emerge from this dark and painful place—because I had to stay strong.

As my husband and I struggled to figure out what to do next, the words of the doctors reverberated in my head. *Don't enable her psychological crutch.* Was it a crutch to help her go to the bathroom? *Nothing real is causing her pain.* I couldn't accept that. The doctors and the PTs didn't see her laboring more and more each day just to accomplish the ordinary tasks of living. They didn't see how much she longed to go to school, be with friends and carry on with her life—and couldn't. They didn't see how much she suffered. But the doctors were right about one thing. More than ever I believed that an insidious invader had taken over my child, and that we had to keep searching for answers. By this point, we'd invested much time and energy in the doctors' perverse combination of tough love, physical therapy, and psychological counseling. Even though we had done everything they'd told us to do, things weren't better. They were markedly worse.

After gut-wrenching discussions, my husband and I finally decided to break with the doctors' advice and rent another wheelchair. Abandoning the plan laid out for us at the hospital and admitting we'd lost faith in so-called experts felt like a point of no return. Looking back, I see it as the pivotal moment when we reclaimed decision-making power for the health and welfare of our child. But at the time, I was awash in conflicting emotions. My heart pounded as I drove to the medical supply store. Was I making a mistake? Were the doctors right? I half-expected somebody from Child Protective Services to jump out of the bushes and arrest me for child abuse.

Getting another wheelchair solved a logistical problem. But what should we do next? It seemed pointless to consult more of the same kinds of doctors, offering more of the same tests and theories. Must we reconcile ourselves to having Rachel imprisoned by pain? I couldn't accept that. Having defied the doctors by getting the wheelchair, I now fiercely embraced what I came to call NSU—no stone unturned. I would find the answers we needed if it took my last breath. But how?

It dawned on me that all the doctors we had seen had operated within the same medical mindset. They read each other's notes and took cues from one another. We needed a fresh pair of eyes—someone to look at it from a different perspective. I tracked down an alternative healer who specializes in acupuncture and herbal remedies. Did he know anything else we could pursue, a rock we hadn't looked under?

He listened intently and suggested I bring Rachel to see him.

Two important things emerged from Rachel's sessions with the acupuncturist. For starters, he asked her if any positions were more comfortable for her than others. She said she had less pain when her back was at an angle, like on a lounge chair. He turned to me and said, "Why not rent her a hospital bed?"

It sounded so reasonable when he said it! Embarrassed to admit the truth, I stammered: "Um, because the physical therapist told us not to...."

He snorted. "That's ridiculous. She can't sleep when she's so uncomfortable. Rent her a bed!"

Second, after asking lots of questions and examining her gently, he turned to me and said, "I think she might have Lyme disease."

I was floored. *Lyme disease?* All the specialists we'd seen had dismissed that idea. They used the negative results of the Lyme tests as proof I was barking up the wrong tree. I'd abandoned that theory a long time ago, because our previous doctors had convinced me it was wildly out of the question.

"Um, the one thing all the specialists we've seen over the past six months have agreed on for sure is that it couldn't possibly be Lyme disease."

He nodded and stroked his beard. "I think there's a good chance it's Lyme disease." Then he turned to me soberly. "I don't know how to help you. I don't even know who to refer you to. You need to find somebody who can diagnosis it and knows how to treat it."

I started researching again with a vengeance. In 2005, there was not a lot of information about Lyme disease on the Internet, and few books about it on Amazon. (Both situations have changed significantly since then.) However, when I stumbled across online patient support groups like *LymeNet* and *CaliforniaLyme*, I hit pay dirt. I dove into the archives of those groups and vacuumed up all the information I could find.

I found out about the medical controversy surrounding Lyme disease, and that few California doctors would even consider the diagnosis. I was told that lab tests like the ones Rachel had been given were unreliable, often saying you don't have it when you do. (That was a shocker for me. All those doctors at two prestigious medical centers had been so quick to dismiss the possibility of Lyme, based on a test that some experts say is no more accurate than a coin toss.) I learned that you need a doctor to consider the whole picture, including your medical history and all of your symptoms, and then make a clinical diagnosis. But, due to strident controversies in the medical world—often called The Lyme Wars—few doctors are willing to do that. However, there are a handful of courageous physicians who diagnose and treat Lyme outside of the medical mainstream, with good results. Our challenge was to find one and get Rachel in the door.

I came across an online article from the *Washington Post* about the famous author Amy Tan. A few years before, out of the blue, she had started having bizarre physical symptoms that kept her from writing her books. None of the many specialists she had consulted could figure out what was wrong. Finally, a doctor in San Francisco diagnosed her with Lyme disease. With treatment, she could resume writing. I called the doctor who was named in the article and found out his waiting list was six months long.

Finally, through connections on *CaliforniaLyme*, I found out about another Lyme specialist, about a two-hour drive from our house. He had a waiting list, too. But then, we got a phone call. There had been a cancellation, for 4 p.m. on the day before Thanksgiving. It was another turning point in our lives, the beginning of unlocking the mystery surrounding Rachel's imprisonment in pain. There would be years of treatment, a variety of therapies, and a steep learning curve for the whole family. But Rachel would get better. The doctor we saw that day was the key to making it happen.

Sandy:

Rachel's story illustrates how mainstream medicine often fails to consider the suffering child and family. Some of these practitioners completely discount the symptoms the child reports, and summarily dismiss the observations of the parents. Doctors often jump to conclusions when they don't have answers. In my psychotherapy practice, I commonly meet families who have experienced misdiagnosis and potentially harmful treatments for conditions their children do not have. My role is to help these families emerge from this rabbit hole, learn how to pursue answers, and move from victim to survivor to thriver.

I am appalled when doctors and hospitals deny the reality of Lyme disease. If they can't find what they consider to be evidence of a physical cause, many conclude the symptoms must be psychological. False diagnosis and the wrong-headed advice that comes with it can thwart the patient's ability to get well. It can ruin the child's life until and unless parents realize that they have been intimidated by the "experts." Only then do they begin to find their way to a sane approach to caring for their child.

Rachel's situation with the hospital is a perfect example. Had Dorothy not continued to search for answers, where would Rachel be today? Without treatment for Lyme and other tick-borne diseases, how much sicker would she have become? Might she be permanently disabled?

It was a circuitous path to my own Lyme diagnosis. In 1984, I started experiencing severe migraine headaches. Over the next six years, I saw several neurologists, including headache experts at major medical centers. Not one of them could help me. As the headaches worsened and became more frequent, I adapted as best I could. I cut back my office hours, giving myself longer breaks between sessions. I relinquished my independence and relied on others to drive me. I no longer hosted family gatherings around the holidays, something I had always enjoyed.

By 1990, the now-continuous headaches left me barely able to function. Sensitive to light and sound, I spent many days lying on the couch in my basement, the darkest room in my house. I passed the time by watching TV shows at a very low volume. When I developed facial paralysis known as Bell's palsy, my doctor tested me for Lyme disease. I was lucky enough to have a positive blood test. I found a Lyme specialist to treat me and began my journey into the world of tick-borne diseases.

To learn more about this illness that had so radically changed my life, I started attending medical conferences. I gained a greater appreciation for how varied and devastating the symptoms of tick-borne diseases can be. Then, in 1991, a particularly troubling teenager was referred to me for psychotherapy. Previously an honors student, Tommy was failing his classes and had become paranoid. The referring professional hoped that I could get to the root of what appeared to be some type of mental illness.

I saw Tommy and his parents for a two-hour initial evaluation. Communication in the family appeared quite good. There was no evidence of mental illness or family dysfunction, and Tommy did not have a history of trauma. Both parents worried about their son's sudden and dramatic decline. Until recently, Tommy had always liked and done well in school. He even had a career goal in mind, not typical of 15 year olds. Because he wanted to be an environmental scientist, Tommy volunteered at a nature center in New York's beautiful

Hudson Valley. That raised a red flag in my mind. Tommy would be exposed to ticks at the nature center. Might that be a factor here?

Over the course of several weeks, I learned more about Tommy's symptoms. He had difficulty sleeping. He was plagued by intrusive thoughts, including the idea that he could never love anyone, including his pet, because anyone he loved would die. He had a hard time concentrating in school and could not retain what he was supposed to learn. His symptoms fit the profile of what I was learning about the psychiatric and cognitive effects of Lyme disease.

Tommy also now refused to attend school, haunted by obsessive thoughts that there was a hate group on campus who wanted to hurt him. To check out the validity of his distress, I contacted a high-level district administrator to find out if he knew of anything like that going on at the school He looked into it and said there appeared to be no basis for Tommy's fears. I was relieved to hear that. However, the more Tommy expressed his paranoid thoughts, the more concerned I became about his mental health.

Tommy appeared to be suffering from a severe mental illness—perhaps schizophrenia or bipolar disorder. These conditions often surface in the late teens. Because of the seriousness of his symptoms, he might have to be admitted to a psychiatric hospital. If he went down that road, he potentially faced a lifelong journey into the land of the mentally ill. But I couldn't help thinking, "What if it's Lyme disease?"

At the next session, I spoke to his mother alone and told her that I wondered if untreated Lyme was causing Tommy's symptoms. She agreed to ask their pediatrician to give her son a Lyme test. It came back negative, and the doctor said Tommy definitely did not have Lyme disease.

I'd only attended a few Lyme conferences at that point, but I knew that lab tests were unreliable. Since the stakes were so high—at this point, Tommy was close to a psychiatric hospital admission—I pushed the envelope. I suggested that his mother take Tommy to a Lyme specialist for a second opinion. She agreed.

After their first visit, the specialist called to tell me he was certain that Tommy had Lyme disease. He did not want to delay treatment while awaiting the results of the blood tests he had sent to a specialty lab. Thus, he made a clinical diagnosis of Lyme disease and prescribed an antibiotic that crossed the blood brain barrier. The doctor hoped that eradicating bacteria in Tommy's brain would clear up the symptoms of a major mental illness.

Indeed, within three days, Tommy's paranoia disappeared completely and he could also now sleep through the night. However, he still had serious issues with Lyme disease, including profound fatigue and disabling leg pain. It took a long time for Tommy to fully recover. But the symptom that almost landed him in a mental hospital—paranoia—was gone after 72 hours of antibiotics. He was spared a life of being mislabeled as mentally ill. If he'd gone down that road, the true cause of his psychiatric symptoms would probably never have been found. Today, the young man who was failing everything at age 15 is a successful attorney with a young family and is in good health.

My experience with Tommy was an eye-opener. Practicing in the highly endemic Hudson Valley, I now had Lyme disease on my professional radar. When I suggested that more of my clients be evaluated for it, many turned out to have Lyme and other tick-borne diseases at the root of their symptoms. Children with eating disorders. Teenagers self-medicating their pain with drugs, alcohol, or self-injury (cutting). Families torn apart by their children's destructive behavior. When Lyme was identified and treated, many of these problems diminished or disappeared.

Getting back to Rachel's story, what was the significant difference between the doctors who concluded that it was not Lyme and the alternative practitioner who thought it might be? The physicians jumped to the "psychological cause" when they failed to find answers. The acupuncturist listened to the patient with an open mind.

Where would Rachel and Tommy be now if their mothers had believed the mainstream physicians and stopped pursuing answers? It takes courage for parents to buck the establishment. Their journey is often a long and lonely one.

two

What Is Lyme Disease, And Why Is It So Controversial?

Families facing the challenges of Lyme disease have a steep learning curve. As they sort out their child's health needs, they must also navigate a political minefield. For a variety of reasons, Lyme is a disputed medical diagnosis. The controversy often prevents people with Lyme from getting effectively treated. However, when parents are looking for answers, they don't know this. Whether they see their trusted local pediatrician or go to a major medical center, they expect to find answers. They don't anticipate getting caught in the middle of a raging medical debate. It's a confusing and distressing place to be.

To understand what they are up against, parents need answers to some basic questions. What is this illness that's holding their family hostage? Why is it so difficult to figure out? Why is practically everything connected with Lyme disease fraught with controversy? Why are some doctors hostile to the very idea of a Lyme diagnosis? And finally, given this unfortunate situation, how can parents find the help their child needs?

Lyme, Ticks, and Diagnostic Uncertainty

Lyme disease is an infection caused by a spirochete, a corkscrew-shaped bacterium called *Borrelia burgdorferi*. It is spread primarily by the bite of *Ixodes* ticks, often called deer ticks. A pregnant woman may also transmit Lyme disease to her unborn baby. Ticks are not insects, but rather tiny, spider-like arachnids, often found in wooded or grassy areas. As a natural part of their life cycle, ticks feed on rodents and other small animals, where they may pick up infections such as Lyme disease. Later they can pass these bacteria along to birds and other animals, including humans.

Ticks tend to stay low to the ground, in leaf litter, grasses, on fallen logs, and tree trunks. They can even be found on the underside of wooden picnic tables. If you brush by them, they may transfer to your shoes or clothing and then crawl around searching for bare skin. When a tick finds its target and inserts its mouth into your body, it secretes a painkilling substance. Thus, you may not feel anything while it is attached. Left undisturbed, the tick might hang on for several days. As it feeds on your blood, it may infect you with any diseases it harbors.

Not all ticks are infected. But those that are can carry many microorganisms, not just the Lyme spirochete. Ticks have four life-stages: egg, larva, nymph, and adult. After hatching, ticks require a blood meal at each stage. As they feed on mice, birds, squirrels, deer, or other wild animals, they may pick up viruses, worms or protozoa, as well as Lyme disease and other bacterial infections. When finished with its blood meal, the tick detaches and falls off. Many times Lyme is transmitted by nymphal ticks, immature ones that are the size of poppy seeds. Because of the tick's tiny size and painless bite, people may not even realize that they have been bitten.

Lyme disease can be a vexing condition to recognize. The most obvious outward sign of early Lyme is a skin lesion called an erythema migrans (EM) rash. It's often described as a bull's eye—a small red ring within a larger red ring. However, studies show that most EM rashes don't look like a Target logo. Most are oval-shaped and solid-colored, with a reddish hue that can range from faint salmon to deep purple. Occasionally, there may be tiny blisters at the edge of the rash. Adding to the confusion, the Centers for Disease Control (CDC) says that in 30 percent of Lyme cases, no rash appears. Thus, relying on an EM rash to diagnose Lyme disease is problematic.

Some newly infected people feel like they have the flu: fever, sore muscles, headaches, and fatigue. Yet others may manifest no early indications at all. When people without any initial signs of the illness eventually develop symptoms—weeks, months, or years after a tick bite—they and their doctors may have no reason to suspect Lyme disease. Missing the window for early diagnosis and treatment allows unrecognized Lyme to spread throughout the body. Once that happens, it is difficult to eradicate.

A person with undiagnosed Lyme might first notice joint pain, gastrointestinal upsets, or migraine-like headaches. Or a variety of other symptoms may suddenly appear. Lyme disease can result in a wide range of neurological disorders, cognitive dysfunction, memory loss, fatigue, pain, psychiatric manifestations, and even potentially fatal heart conditions. In children, Lyme can also trigger learning disabilities or behavioral problems. Furthermore, co-infections—additional illnesses transmitted by ticks along with Lyme—can cause or intensify both physical and psychiatric symptoms.

Lyme disease is easiest to treat in its early phase. Ideally, our medical system would be set up to identify and treat it as early as possible. This would save individuals the misery of an entrenched illness, reduce medical costs, and allow people to work, pay taxes, and care for their families. Children would be well enough to attend school and less likely to need special education services. Unfortunately, for too many people, the system does not work that way. Instead, the Lyme controversy prevents many infected people from getting the care they need.

The Lyme Wars

There is strong debate about every aspect of Lyme disease: how to define, recognize, and treat the illness, as well as how to identify the number of people who have it. These divisions have given rise to what is sometimes called "The Lyme Wars." Here are some examples of children who have been casualties of the conflict:

- A 10-year-old girl from San Francisco developed a swollen, painful knee. Doctors said she had juvenile rheumatoid arthritis, even though her case didn't fit the JRA profile. Treatment didn't help. Other baffling, disabling symptoms emerged as well. Too disabled to leave the house, she missed most of high school.

- A seven-year-old girl from Maine fell ill with fevers, rashes, and aching joints. She couldn't stay awake at school. She had to give up the dance lessons that she loved. As her doctors treated her for rheumatoid arthritis, her health continued to decline. Neurological symptoms set in, and she lost her ability to read and write.

- A 14-year-old Florida boy experienced spots in his vision, panic attacks, and obsessive thoughts of death. He went from being a happy child to a brooding teenager. He saw ten different doctors, including ophthalmologists, psychologists and infectious disease specialists. None could explain his crushing anxiety, his eye problems, or the complete change in his personality.

- A 4-year-old boy from British Columbia complained about headaches, foot pain, and sore knees. The doctor blamed the knee and foot problems on "growing pains." He attributed the headaches to stress from the child's reaction to his parents' divorce. The pain continued for years. When the boy was 11, his doctors decided he had somatoform disorder and advised psychiatric help. ("Somatoform disorder," a mental illness, assumes there is no physical basis for the pain. In the DSM-5, published in 2015, it is referred to as Somatic Symptom Disorder— see Chapter Six.)

These young people—of different ages, from different parts of the continent—were all eventually found to have Lyme disease. Yet, before that happened, they suffered for years without an accurate diagnosis or appropriate treatment. Some doctors even said they were faking or overstating their symptoms. As a result, they languished for years, ill and isolated, missing out on sports, schooling, and friendships.

Why such uncertainty? First, there is no definitive "gold standard" laboratory test for Lyme disease. Available tests look for antibodies to the Lyme spirochete, not the spirochete itself. Indirect tests of infection often produce negative results. Some studies indicate that the CDC's testing protocol produces false negatives 50 percent of the time. Yet, many physicians assume that a negative result is definitive and at that point they no longer consider Lyme disease as a possibility. (See Chapter Three for a more thorough discussion of testing.)

At this point, it's important to understand how sharply the issue of Lyme disease has divided the medical world. One side is led by the Infectious Diseases Society of America (IDSA), an influential and powerful professional organization made up of doctors and researchers. Although the IDSA is a private association, its guidelines for diagnosing and treating Lyme disease are endorsed by the CDC, and thus are often mistakenly viewed as national policy. The IDSA Lyme guidelines profoundly influence how doctors diagnose and treat the disease, as well as whether or not insurance companies will pay for Lyme-related care. Furthermore, in some states, medical boards have investigated—and occasionally revoked the licenses of—physicians who don't follow the IDSA Lyme guidelines.

The IDSA defines Lyme disease narrowly. According to its guidelines, diagnosis requires either a doctor-confirmed EM rash or positive test results, coupled with a specific set of symptoms. Patients who fall outside of these restrictions will typically be told they do not have Lyme disease, regardless of their symptoms or history of tick bites. For patients who do meet the IDSA's diagnostic standard, the guidelines say that two-to-four-weeks of antibiotic treatment is sufficient to clear the infection. The IDSA says that Lyme disease cannot persist in the body after a short course of antibiotic treatment and denies the existence of chronic Lyme.

Unfortunately, this one-size-fits-all definition of Lyme disease puts patients in a bad spot. If they don't have an EM rash and receive test results that are falsely negative, they are denied access to early treatment—when it's likely to be most effective. And even those who "qualify" for the IDSA's short course of antibiotics may still be symptomatic after finishing their pills. The IDSA does not consider these symptoms to be evidence of chronic Lyme, but rather what it calls "post-treatment Lyme syndrome," for which it offers no remedy. Because most doctors, hospitals, and insurance companies follow the IDSA's lead, such patients are typically refused additional treatment. Patients are on their own to search for further medical help. If they do manage to find a doctor willing to take them on, they may have to travel a long distance and pay out of pocket for treatment.

Here's where the other side of the debate comes in. The International Lyme and Associated Diseases Society (ILADS) represents doctors and researchers who take a broader view of Lyme disease than the IDSA and the CDC. These practitioners assert that Lyme requires a clinical diagnosis, including careful evaluation of a patient's medical history and likely exposure to ticks, a comprehensive physical examination, and ruling out other medical conditions that might be causing the symptoms. Testing is used to complete the picture, but is not the sole basis for establishing or excluding a Lyme diagnosis.

The largest difference between the two groups involves the question of whether or not Lyme spirochetes can persist in the body after a short course of antibiotics, causing a chronic condition that may require longer treatment. The IDSA says there's no such thing as chronic Lyme disease, and that further treatment is wrongheaded and potentially harmful. ILADS practitioners disagree. They point to scientific studies supporting the existence of chronic infection, as well as a large body of clinical evidence showing that many patients recover after longer treatment.

The Lyme patient community has come to refer to ILADS-affiliated doctors as "Lyme-literate," often abbreviated as LLMD. While the term is imprecise, it generally describes a physician with in-depth knowledge of Lyme disease, co-infections, and other conditions that often accompany or exacerbate the illness. Most LLMDs regularly attend ILADS' annual medical conferences to learn from other clinicians who are diagnosing and treating Lyme, and to enrich their understanding of tick-borne diseases by networking with their colleagues.

Advocates have long argued that the IDSA guidelines deny access to proper medical care to people with Lyme disease. In 2008, then-Connecticut Attorney General Richard Blumenthal (now a U.S. Senator) completed a civil investigation of the IDSA's 2006 Lyme guidelines and said the organization's guidelines process was "flawed." In a press release, he stated:

My office uncovered undisclosed financial interests held by several of the most powerful IDSA panelists. The IDSA's guideline panel improperly ignored or minimized consideration of alternative medical opinion and evidence regarding chronic Lyme disease, potentially raising serious questions about whether the recommendations reflected all relevant science.

At the time, Lyme advocates hoped Blumenthal's finding would lead to revamping of the troublesome guidelines. That did not happen, however, and the IDSA Lyme guidelines remain in force. (As this book goes to press in 2015, the IDSA is reviewing its Lyme disease guidelines. Will this improve things for Lyme patients? We're not holding our breath. See LymeDisease.org's website for continuing updates about the process.)

There is also vast disagreement about how many people have Lyme disease. This matters, because public health resources tend to go towards illnesses perceived as affecting a large part of the population. If Lyme disease is not seen as a significant threat to public health, lawmakers won't spend tax money to combat it, local health departments won't educate the public about tick bite prevention, and schools won't consider the need to provide special services to students with Lyme.

Another obstacle to reliable counting of cases involves how individual states report Lyme figures to the federal government. Because different regions use different criteria to track the disease, the CDC receives numbers that are not statistically comparable. To avoid this "apples and oranges" situation, the agency only tabulates cases that meet its strict case definition. All others are rejected.

For instance, if a particular case was diagnosed on the basis of an EM rash, the CDC only accepts it if a doctor has verified that the rash was at least five centimeters in diameter. A case with a known tick bite, Lyme symptoms, and a physician-confirmed EM rash of 4.5 centimeters is left out. Other ways to qualify a case require layers of paperwork that some localities find too burdensome to pursue. Journalist Mary Beth Pfeiffer writes in the *Poughkeepsie Journal*:

> *Eighteen New York counties, including all in the mid-Hudson region, save staff time and money by not having to follow up with physicians on every reported Lyme case; instead, they estimate cases using a complex formula that counts cases with the distinctive Lyme rash and extrapolates the rest from a random sample. But that means thousands of cases cannot be submitted to the federal government.*

The *Poughkeepsie Journal* is located in an area with one of the highest number of Lyme disease cases in the country.

For the past several years, the CDC has reported about 30,000 Lyme cases per year across the nation—the number of state-submitted cases that met its strict surveillance criteria. However, in August 2013, the CDC increased its annual estimate of diagnosed Lyme cases to 300,000 per year. The agency based the higher number on three studies that each used different methods for arriving at an estimate. In a press release, the CDC's Dr. Paul Mead stated:

> *We know that routine surveillance only gives us part of the picture, and that the true number of illnesses is much greater...This new preliminary estimate confirms that Lyme disease is a tremendous public health problem in the United States, and clearly highlights the urgent need for prevention*.

27

Based on statistical analysis of past reporting patterns, some experts estimate that the actual number of new cases could be well over a million per year.

Reporting discrepancies, undercounting, and less-than-definitive testing all contribute to widespread under-acknowledgement of Lyme disease. The fact that physicians risk losing their licenses if they treat Lyme disease makes the situation even grimmer. This seems to be a factor in what many patients experience as "Lyme blindness" in the medical world. People who actually have Lyme disease are routinely told they couldn't possibly have it. This puts parents of sick children in a terrible bind.

What Are Parents to Do?

Ann Corson, MD, is an integrative family physician from Pennsylvania. In the Summer 2006 issue of *The Lyme Times*, she describes how she found out firsthand what parents go through.

> *When my only child was 14, we moved to Chester County, PA. We had no understanding of the dangers of ticks or of their prevalence in our new surroundings. My son came to me one night with an engorged deer tick on his left ear. I removed it carefully and cleansed the area. Then, as I had been taught, I did not treat but watched and waited for signs of disease. If only I had known the consequences of that one tick bite. If only I had known that I could send that fat juicy tick off to a lab to check for the presence of four different tick-borne diseases. Watchful waiting only allowed the nightmare of illness to grow.*

> *My son never had a flu-like illness or an EM rash. He just became ill insidiously over many months with a sore throat here, a headache there, and with lots of abdominal pain. I took him for second opinions and was told more than once that nothing was seriously wrong, that he had irritable bowel syndrome or emotional problems.*

Over the next two years, as her son's health worsened, he had three negative tests for Lyme disease. Eventually, he was bedbound and unable to function. Then, Corson writes, a friend handed her a Lyme information pamphlet, which opened her eyes to a different approach to diagnosing tick-borne diseases. Subsequent evaluations and different testing confirmed that her son indeed had Lyme, as well as the co-infections Babesia, Bartonella, and Mycoplasma fermentans. In time, comprehensive treatment brought improvement. Corson's son went on to graduate from college and become an independent adult.

In recent years, blogs and other social media convey countless similar experiences. In a YouTube video, a Wisconsin mother speaks about her previously active daughter, whose health took a nosedive at age 13. None of the many doctors they consulted helped in any way.

She couldn't talk, she couldn't walk, she used a wheelchair. She resembled someone with Parkinson's. Her eyes blinked rapidly. She had a lot of motor tics and uncontrollable jerking motions. Most of the time she spent lying on the floor in a seizure-like episode, with her hands clenched, and drooling. Other parts of the day she was just vacant and stared at a wall, not really aware of what was going on. It was devastating for our whole family to watch our daughter fall apart before our eyes.

This family eventually found a doctor who understood that this was a complex manifestation of Lyme disease and began treatment. After 18 months of IV antibiotics, the teenager improved enough to leave her wheelchair behind and walk with canes. However, she still has significant health issues and continues treatment.

A Florida mother says it took a year for her son to get properly diagnosed with Lyme disease. Their first inkling of a problem came when her 11-year-old boy started complaining of dizziness. As the child's condition rapidly declined, none of their doctors could figure out why.

My son suffered excruciating pain, missed half of sixth grade, was fainting, and lost the ability to walk on many days. Sometimes he had migraines that required IV morphine. He would be screaming for help. It was brutal.

When the mother asked if could possibly be Lyme disease, doctors told her "Lyme does not exist in Florida." Eventually, the family found a doctor who recognized that her son had Lyme disease and six other infections. She believes the delay in diagnosis contributed to the severity of her son's illness.

As these young people and their families found out the hard way, they had to wage a battle on two fronts. While dealing with the physical and mental symptoms of Lyme disease, they also had to fight for proper medical treatment. Some of these children were misdiagnosed and treated for illnesses they did not have. Others were denied treatment altogether. In addition, the infrastructure for dealing with a catastrophically ill child—medical care, insurance coverage, educational accommodations, social services—was not on their side.

Gestational Lyme Disease

There is another aspect to this controversy that gets little attention. It is gestational Lyme disease—when an infected mother transmits the pathogen to her unborn child. Dr. Charles Ray Jones, a Connecticut pediatrician who has treated more than 15,000 children with Lyme disease, has documented hundreds of cases of children who were born with the illness. In his experience, these children can display a wide range of symptoms. These often include hypotonia ("floppy baby syndrome"), developmental delays, learning disabilities, pain, fatigue, low-grade fevers, vomiting, ear infections, and eye problems as well as noise, light, and skin sensitivity. Many of them improve dramatically with Lyme disease treatment.

The CDC views pregnancy-related Lyme disease differently, stating on its website:

> *Lyme disease acquired during pregnancy may lead to infection of the placenta and possible stillbirth; however, **no negative effects on the fetus have been found when the mother receives appropriate antibiotic treatment.** (bold type added by authors.)*

Unfortunately, because unreliable testing makes it difficult for anybody—pregnant or not—to get diagnosed and treated in a timely manner, we believe the CDC should do more to inform doctors and the general public about Lyme-related risks of pregnancy.

Regardless of whether children became infected before or after birth, their parents have a tough row to hoe. They must search for answers while earning a living, running a household and meeting the needs of other family members. They must also deal with medical and educational systems that may conflict with their child's best interests. Parents must do Internet research, marshal resources and figure out a plan of action on their own. The process is confusing, expensive, and difficult.

three

Searching For Answers

Dorothy:

MOST PEOPLE WITH A SICK CHILD take her to the family doctor. That's what we did when my daughter first became ill. And it's what I'd expect anybody else to do in a similar situation. But, if your child has Lyme disease and co-infections, you probably won't hear about that from your family doctor. Instead, you may find yourself on a forced march from primary care offices to various medical specialties. There will be stops along the way for blood draws, X-rays or other procedures. (A survey by LymeDisease.org found that most patients consult at least seven doctors before receiving a Lyme diagnosis. A third of them see 10 or more.)

Throughout this process, you still have to deal with on-going work and family obligations. You must care for your suffering child, manage medical appointments, and do your best to get through each day. You may be referred to a specialist, with a waiting list of six weeks or more. Perhaps that doctor then refers you to another specialist, also with a waiting list. This can drag on for months.

In the early days of my daughter's illness, Rachel's major symptom was intense, body-wide pain. Her knees and ankles hurt

32

too much for her to put any weight on them at all, so the only way she could get around was by wheelchair. Also, her shoulders and upper back were so hypersensitive, that even a feather-light touch to that area was extremely painful. Yet, the doctors we saw had no answers, and we remained in limbo, waiting for the next medical appointment and then the next, and the next.

Only parts of our home were wheelchair accessible. Getting in and out of the house was manageable, but the wheelchair couldn't navigate our narrow carpeted hallway and small bathroom. One day in exasperation, I hired someone to rip out the carpet and put vinyl flooring in the hall and Rachel's bedroom. Then, we used a smaller, wheeled office chair to push her from her bedroom to the bathroom. This single action tangibly improved our day-to-day lives.

With about six weeks until the end of the school year, Rachel wanted to complete seventh grade. Typically, I'd push her wheelchair the few blocks to school and deposit her at her first classroom. Later, one of her pals would push her wheelchair from class to class. Sometimes, Rachel missed school for medical appointments. Other times, the pain was too much and she stayed home. But mostly, she went to school to see friends, keep up with her studies, and do something besides wallow in misery and isolation.

It was a bizarre and frightening time. With our pediatrician on maternity leave, we didn't have a specific doctor managing our case. And once other doctors in the medical group referred us to specialists, they didn't want to deal with us at all. I even had difficulty persuading a doctor to sign off on a required medical excuse for physical education class.

"But she's in constant pain and in a wheelchair," I said to the young female doctor who hesitated to sign the PE waiver. "She can't do PE."

The doctor looked at me sharply. "We didn't prescribe that wheelchair. You got it on your own." The disapproval in her voice was palpable.

It was a theme doctors came back to, time and again. They faulted me profoundly for "putting my daughter in a wheelchair." They said that was clear evidence that I "wanted" her to be sick and disabled. Huh? I wanted to get her from Point A to Point B, and I didn't know how else to do that, seeing as she couldn't walk. The doctor reluctantly signed the PE waiver. Then she brusquely told me not to contact her again until after we'd seen the specialist.

In the meantime, a serious incident happened at school that I knew nothing about. It involved another seventh grader whom I will call Anita. For some reason, seeing Rachel in a wheelchair set Anita on a warpath. The girl started quietly heckling Rachel. She'd walk by, whisper an obscenity and keep going. Soon, Anita apparently recruited followers—both boys and girls—to do the same thing. They'd walk up to Rachel with a smile, mutter something obnoxious and move on.

One day, as Rachel's friend pushed her to class, Anita materialized in front of them. "You think you're so great because you're in a wheelchair," she taunted, peppering the comment with profanity. "You think you're better than everybody else." Then Anita grabbed a pile of books and notes from Rachel's lap, flung them towards a trash can and departed. Hurt, angry and embarrassed, Rachel burst into tears. Her friend scrambled after the papers fluttering in the breeze and then took Rachel to the school office. Both girls were crying.

A staff member listened to Rachel and her friend, and then called in Anita. Surprisingly, her story pretty much matched Rachel's. Yes, she had thrown Rachel's books and papers. No, Rachel hadn't said or done anything to her. She added: "Rachel sits in that wheelchair like she's better than everybody else. It just makes me mad!"

The staff member advised the girls to find a way to work it out and sent them back to class. Because the school never notified me of what had happened and Rachel kept it to herself, I was unaware that this upsetting event had made Rachel's life even more difficult. It would be months before Rachel told my husband and me what had happened. When I called the school at that late date and asked why I hadn't been contacted, I was told: "We find it's better if students handle such problems on their own." (The issue of school bullying had not achieved media prominence in 2005. I wonder if junior high staff would take the same position today.)

School employees and unfriendly classmates weren't the only ones with little empathy for a young girl in pain. As we continued on our merry-go-round of medical appointments, I noticed a disturbing pattern. Each time we saw a new practitioner, the conversation went something like this:

Nurse: "Please rate your pain on a scale of one to ten. One is hardly any pain at all and ten is the worst pain you can imagine."

Rachel, with no hesitation: "Ten."

Nurse (smiling and shaking her head): "Oh, no, dear. You don't understand. It's not a ten. You're not in that much pain. Ten is the *worst pain you can possibly imagine.*"

Rachel, with no hesitation: "Ten."

Nurse, sighing: "I'll put down an eight." Then she leaves the room.

It soon became obvious that this was a pervasive mindset. The practitioners had a mental image of what ten-out-of-ten pain looked like, and Rachel didn't match it. To them (kind of like Anita at the junior high school) she just looked like a normal girl sitting in a wheelchair. Because at that moment she wasn't howling in anguish, she couldn't possibly have excruciating pain. (One nurse said, "No dear, number ten pain would be at least equal to childbirth." As if my 13-year-old daughter had a frame of reference for that.)

Part of the problem was how they phrased it. They always said, "Ten is the worst you can imagine." I once pointed out that maybe this *was* the worst Rachel could imagine. The nurse glared at me and said, "Let her answer for herself."

I wanted to cry out to every medical person we saw: *She feels like she's being stung by bees! We have to push her on a rolling office chair to get to the bathroom. Sometimes her foot feels like it's on fire.* But they just seemed to want a data point for their chart.

Children with Lyme disease may experience many different kinds of pain. It can be difficult to figure out what's causing it. Many of them hurt for years, with little help or understanding from the medical system. And because children may not be adept at describing their pain, it is often underestimated.

Here's what one mother said about a daughter whose symptoms began at age 5:

> *I was told that the eye pain was because she was in kindergarten and starting to read, the joint pain was growing pains, and the fatigue was just her talking and getting attention or being lazy, and she needed more exercise.*

Three years later, the girl's symptoms and pain intensified.

> *They mentioned psychiatric stuff and took her in a separate room to ask if this was attention-getting because maybe she had been molested (their theory). They said to wear supportive shoes. They gave her no good pain meds. They offered ibuprofen.... She was supposed to go to a special study for children with inexplicable pain (since she absolutely positively could not possibly have Lyme, because it "doesn't exist" in California) but somehow that never happened.*

A New York mother recounts that her child, whom I will call Becky, began to experience leg pain when she was 2 or 3 years old.

> *By age 6, Becky suffered from lots of muscle and joint pain, headaches, stomach aches...She was often unable to walk due to the pain in her legs and the extreme weakness that would hit. I got her crutches, which helped some when she needed them. At times she would be walking along the room and then just melt into the floor and scoot on her bottom to get to where she was going.*

As the pain continued for years, her mother reports, Becky hated being asked to rate it on the one to ten scale. "She never really knew a life without pain. So it was difficult to rate something as none-to-horrible when all you knew was moderate-to-horrible." Finally, at age 14, Becky was diagnosed and treated for Lyme disease and her pain reduced significantly.

Lyme disease is named after Lyme, Connecticut, where it was first recognized in the 1970s. The area continues to be a hotbed for the infection. So, it shouldn't be a stretch for a doctor in that state to suspect Lyme disease in a sick child, especially when there's a known tick bite. Yet, that is not the experience of many families.

A Connecticut mother tells of her 3-year-old boy, who had been bitten by a tick. Soon, he experienced knee pain, rashes, and fevers that would come and go. "Because we had gotten the tick out right away and it wasn't engorged, we were told it couldn't possibly be Lyme disease."

The knee pain worsened. He no longer wanted to run and play, but rather sat listlessly all day. The mother pushed to have him evaluated for Lyme disease, but the doctors dismissed her concerns. When their son was still in pain nine months after the tick bite, the family finally took him to a physician more familiar with Lyme disease. This doctor found that the child indeed had Lyme. Antibiotic therapy has relieved many of the symptoms, though at this writing, treatment is on-going.

At this stage of the game, when a child is suffering and the doctors aren't helping, it's common for a parent to doubt herself. Am I doing everything I can to help my child? Is there something I've overlooked? God forbid, is this somehow my fault? Unfortunately, the medical establishment often creates or feeds these doubts. The mother is usually the one who is most engaged with the afflicted child. She shares those sleepless nights, witnesses firsthand the child's anguish, and shuffles the youngster to medical appointments, yet, her ideas about what might be going on are often dismissed by the so-called experts. They may say she is "overly engaged" with her child's health problems. Or, like in my case, that I somehow "wanted" my daughter in a wheelchair.

At one point, before we knew what was wrong with Rachel, I made an appointment to see a counselor myself. The stress of her deteriorating condition was taking a toll on me, too, and I needed help holding things together. The therapist told me flat out that I spent too much time thinking about my daughter's health. She said I needed to develop other interests. At the time, I was too flummoxed to respond. But here's my response: "What if my child was trapped inside a house that was on fire, and I was trying to get her out? Would you say I was 'overly engaged' with her welfare? Would you say I should stop trying to save her and find myself a hobby?" Lyme-related catastrophic illness is like a house on fire. Families need help battling the flames and rescuing their children.

What Are Your Child's Symptoms?

Because children who are sick may not be very good at describing how they feel, parents need to observe them closely to figure out what's going on. Does your child complain of headaches or stomachaches? Is she more irritable than usual? Is he unable to sleep well at night? Are there problems at school? Have there been outbursts and mood swings? Has the child lost interest in activities she used to enjoy? These important clues might or might not indicate Lyme disease. It's vital that you—and your doctor—consider all factors that might be contributing to these symptoms.

Thus, it's important for parents to understand the concept of "differential diagnosis." This is the process a physician uses to distinguish between conditions with similar symptoms. For example, let's say a patient has pain in the abdomen. The doctor may suspect appendicitis, but he still needs to rule out other possibilities, such as food poisoning or kidney stones.

Unfortunately, many physicians don't include Lyme disease in their differential diagnoses. Patients may go from doctor to doctor, searching for answers for years, without Lyme even being considered. Other times, based on an unreliable diagnostic test, Lyme may be mistakenly ruled out. If your child has continuing, unexplained medical problems, take action. Find someone who will properly evaluate him for Lyme and other tick-borne diseases, as well as for anything else that might be contributing to the symptoms. Of course, that's easier said than done. How does a parent even begin the process of looking? Persistence and a good Internet connection can help.

You need to educate yourself about the complexities of Lyme disease. The following websites and books are a good place to start. More are listed in Appendix A.

- www.lymedisease.org
- www.lymefamilies.com
- www.ilads.org

- www.childrenslymenetwork.org
- *The Beginner's Guide to Lyme Disease,* by Dr. Nicola McFadzean
- *Coping with Lyme Disease: A Practical Guide to Dealing with Diagnosis and Treatment,* by Denise Lang, with Kenneth Liegner, MD

As you research, I recommend joining at least one support group, either in-person or online. Such groups can offer tangible help, such as doctor recommendations, as well as emotional support from others who are traveling a similar path. Online groups, especially, are very diverse. Some groups are open to anybody (Lymenet.org). Others are geographically based (CaliforniaLyme, NewYorkLyme, etc.) or focused by narrower interest (LymeParents, Lyme and Pregnancy). Some are on freestanding websites, while others are on social media platforms, such as Facebook and LinkedIn. (See appendix for more information.) Dealing with the challenges of Lyme disease can be a lonely experience. A community of people who share your concerns can help cut through that isolation.

Don't be intimidated by doctors who discourage you from finding information or support online. A physician who tells you to "leave it to the experts," may not be a good fit. Look for someone willing to see you as a partner in helping your child get well, someone who will respond to your questions and concerns.

When you finally find a doctor who is willing to explore Lyme disease as a possible source of your child's problems, what can you reasonably expect to happen? For starters, the doctor should review your child's complete medical history. This should include the mother's history, as well. How was her health at conception? Was it a complicated pregnancy? Did she have a known tick bite and/or tick-borne diseases? The physician should perform a detailed physical examination and order appropriate tests for Lyme, as well as anything else that might be triggering the child's current medical problems. The goal should be to get a complete picture of the patient's health. In *The Beginner's Guide to Lyme Disease*, Nicola McFadzean ND, observes

> *The key concept to grasp here is that of underlying cause.... Many disease pictures with varying symptoms may be thought to be different diseases because they have different symptoms, when in fact the underlying cause may be singular: Lyme disease.*

Lyme Disease Symptom Overview

The following list of Lyme disease symptoms in children is re-printed by permission from the website of the Children's Lyme Disease Network, to which pediatrician Charles Ray Jones, MD, is an advisor. Dr. Jones describes some of the most common symptoms he has seen in his 40-plus years of clinical experience treating more than 15,000 pediatric patients suffering from Lyme disease and associated tick-transmitted illnesses.

- **Fatigue.** This symptom is universal in children with Lyme disease. Fatigue can be intermittent or ongoing. Or a child may suddenly have poor stamina, unable to perform physical activities they once enjoyed. A child can be energetic and then collapse or 'wilt' from exhaustion, or they can be completely bedridden with fatigue.

  For example: A 4-year-old patient would run on the playground with other kids but needed to sit down after only a few minutes. This patient wasn't sleeping all day, but he did not have the stamina that a healthy 4-year-old should have. Another 14-year-old patient experienced fatigue so extreme that spending a few hours out with his friends after school would land him in bed for several days just recuperating.

- **Joint pain.** Migratory joint pain is a hallmark of Lyme disease. The pain can travel between different joints or the intensity of pain may vary for the affected joints. Typically, more than one joint is involved. Larger joints are usually impacted, including the knees, hips, shoulders, and elbows. The knee joints may be painful but do not have to be swollen. Pain can also occur in smaller joints, like the fingers, wrists, hands, ankles, and feet. There may also be pain in the child's neck and back.

  Young children can have difficulty describing their pain. Continuously rubbing and massaging an affected joint may be an indication that a child is having joint pain. The pain can also stop a child from doing a particular activity. *For example: A patient would become oppositional when asked to cross his legs while sitting on the floor during reading hour in his pre-K class. The teacher complained to the parents. When questioned, the patient explained that his knees felt better when his legs were straight.*

- **Muscle pain and weakness.** Muscle pain is often generalized and usually does not have a trigger point location. Children may have morning stiffness, and muscle weakness that will impact their ability to play sports or physical activities. They may experience muscle stiffness and pain in their neck and upper back. Some patients are unable to walk or stand due to muscle weakness. *For example: Some children are unable to walk or stand due to extreme muscle weakness. One young patient had difficulty walking. The parents were told their child needed to see a* *psychiatrist. I diagnosed him with Lyme disease. He was treated and today is running around with his other siblings.*

- **Migraine and non-migraine headaches.** Young children often describe their headaches as a general soreness or pressure on their head.

  For example: Young patients have described headaches by saying their "hair hurts" or by holding their head. Some patients will gently press their head up against an object or person, trying to relieve the pain.

- **Fevers and night sweats.** Fevers are usually low grade and can be associated with chills. A low-grade fever for a young child can be anywhere between 99°F and 101°F.

- **Sleep disturbances.** A child may be sleeping too much or may have difficulty falling asleep. He may have night terrors, bedtime fears, and anxiety.

- **Gastrointestinal pain.** Stomach pain, including nausea and other digestive issues, may be present.

- **Urinary problems.** A child may have pain when urinating, urinate more frequently, or may develop urinary incontinence.

- **Irritability and impulsivity.** Children may have a low frustration tolerance and difficulty focusing. Schoolwork can suffer.

  For example: Patients have been misdiagnosed with attention deficit hyperactivity disorder (ADHD) or oppositional defiant disorder (ODD). When treated appropriately with antibiotics, these behaviors have disappeared.

- **Mood swings, emotional liability.** Children may exhibit uncharacteristic and/or abrupt personality changes. They may appear depressed or anxious.

- **Obsessive-compulsive behaviors.** OCD-type behaviors may be present. Compulsions might be hard to recognize in toddlers and young children. Compulsions can be subtle.

  For example: A patient may have a compulsion with chewing or touching things. Turning on and off light switches, continuously touching objects around them.

  A 3-year-old patient would chew on his shirt collar incessantly but the mother didn't recognize something was wrong until he chewed a hole through a young girl's stockings while they were resting during nap time.

- **Bursts of aggression/rage.** Parents will say their child changed overnight and became a different kid. They'll display behavior outbursts or mood swings that are uncharacteristic. This behavioral change is also described in patients diagnosed with PANS or PANDAS. [Note from authors: more on this later in the chapter.]

- **Brain fog.** This is frequently reported. Children may suddenly be more forgetful. Their short-term memory may be poor, or they can have difficulty in processing information. They don't think as fast as they used to.

  For example: A child, who is having trouble processing information, may have difficulty with word finding and will repeat the same word several times, while searching to retrieve the next word. This may be confused with stuttering.

- **Light, sound, touch, and taste sensitivity.** A child may be extremely sensitive to lights, sounds, touch or tastes. Everyday sounds, like noise from a television or sounds in the school cafeteria, can make the child uncomfortable. He may become angry when touched. This sensitivity is more than being fussy. It will interfere with the child's daily life.

For example: One patient was so sensitive to touch that she couldn't hug her parents. Another patient had to wear sunglasses inside the house, even when all the blinds and curtains were closed.

According to Dr. Jones, children can be very sick with Lyme and not meet any of the CDC criteria for official recognition of their condition. Furthermore, he points out that because Lyme can affect systems throughout the whole body, it can be hard to parse out which symptoms are specifically due to Lyme and which are not.

Teenagers

Because Lyme can affect hormone levels in the body, teenagers may have symptoms not seen in younger children. Adolescent girls might experience pelvic pain, menstrual problems, or ovarian cysts. They might have mood swings around the time of their menstrual periods. Boys may have testicular pain, as well as low testosterone levels, which can contribute to fatigue and inadequate physical development. Both girls and boys can manifest anxiety, depression, and self-mutilating behaviors. They might self-medicate with alcohol or illicit drugs. Oblivious to these physical symptoms, parents may attribute behavior problems to adolescent rebelliousness or even to a psychiatric disorder.

Other Tick-Borne Diseases

When Lyme-literate practitioners refer to Lyme disease, they typically mean Lyme and a whole complex of other tick-borne illnesses. "Ticks are cesspools of disease," says Dr. Ann Corson, and can transmit several pathogens at once. She says 80 percent of her pediatric Lyme patients have at least one co-infection. She notes that co-infected patients are sicker and require longer treatment in order to get well. Some people get multiple infections from a single tick bite. Others may get bitten by various ticks at more or less the same time. For example, a child who jumps in a pile of leaves and rolls around on the ground may pick up different kinds of ticks, which could potentially carry separate diseases.

There are more than a dozen known tick-borne infections in addition to Lyme (*Borrelia burgdorferi*). Here are a few of the most common ones:

- **Babesiosis (or babesia)** is caused by a malaria-like parasite that infects red blood cells. Some people with babesiosis show no symptoms. Others may have fever, chills, sweats, headache, unexplained cough or "air hunger" (difficulty in taking a breath.) In the United States, the Northeast and upper Midwest have a very high rate of ticks co-infected with Lyme and babesia. Babesia is most commonly spread by ticks, though it can also be transmitted by contaminated blood transfusions, or from an infected mother to her unborn child.

- **Ehrlichiosis**, carried by the lone star tick, infects the white blood cells. Common manifestations are high fever, severe headaches, flulike symptoms, muscle pain, and fatigue. Sometimes, especially in children, it can cause a rash.

- **Anaplasmosis**, carried by the same kind of ticks that carry Lyme disease, can cause similar symptoms as ehrlichiosis.

- There are many different species of **Bartonella**, some of which can be transmitted by ticks, fleas, and lice, among other vectors. One species, *Bartonella henslae*, can also be spread by cat scratches, and is often called "cat scratch disease." While some forms of Bartonella are mild and self-limiting, others cause serious illness. Bartonella can bring central nervous system irritability, such as tremors and agitation, as well as anxiety, mood swings, obsessive-compulsive disorder, and anti-social behavior. Often, Bartonella is accompanied by a skin rash that may look like stretch marks.

Other tick-borne diseases include Colorado tick fever virus, Powassan encephalitis virus, Q Fever, Rocky Mountain spotted fever (Rickettsia), tick-borne relapsing fever (*Borrelia hermsii* and *Borrelia miyamotoi*), tularemia, and brucellosis. The fact that Lyme disease can coexist with other infections is one reason it can be so difficult to sort out and treat. Furthermore, other factors complicate the picture even more.

In his groundbreaking book, *Why Can't I Get Better? Solving the Mystery of Lyme and Chronic Disease*, Dr. Richard Horowitz states:

> *Instead of looking for one answer, I believe we should be looking for many. The majority of my Lyme patients, as well as others suffering from persistent chronic illness, generally do not have one sole cause for their symptoms. They often have an overlapping set of medical problems.*

Horowitz primarily treats adults. However, his perspective can be useful in evaluating children as well. He offers a new way of looking at Lyme and chronic illness. He calls it multiple systemic infectious disease syndrome, or MSIDS. He recommends the following 16-point diagnostic tool to help uncover the root cause of symptoms.

MSIDS: Overlapping Factors Contributing to Chronic Illness
1. Lyme disease and co-infections
2. Immune dysfunction

3. Inflammation
4. Environmental toxins
5. Functional medicine abnormalities with nutritional deficiencies
6. Mitochondrial dysfunction
7. Endocrine abnormalities
8. Neurodegenerative disorders
9. Neuropsychiatric disorders
10. Sleep disorders
11. Autonomic nervous system dysfunction and POTS
12. Allergies
13. Gastrointestinal disorders
14. Liver dysfunction
15. Pain disorders/addiction
16. Lack of exercise/deconditioning

In correspondence with the authors, Dr. Horowitz expands on number 11, regarding autonomic nervous system dysfunction and Postural Orthostatic Tachycardia Syndrome, also known as POTS. Dr. Horowitz says the autonomic nervous system, which controls our blood pressure, pulse rate, bowel and bladder function, is frequently affected by Lyme. He notes that children with POTS may have episodes of dizziness, fainting, and difficulty standing for long periods of time. They may have fast heartbeats, palpitations, brain fog, and problems with bladder and bowel function. During an evaluation for POTS, Dr. Horowitz advises taking the child's blood pressure and pulse rates at different intervals (at 0, 5, and 10 minutes) while both sitting and standing. He also recommends a tilt table test, which monitors symptoms while the patient is held in different positions (from lying flat to standing up straight).

In his book and on his website (www.cangetbetter.com), Dr. Horowitz offers a detailed Lyme-MSIDS symptom questionnaire. The questionnaire has been statistically validated by researchers at State University of New York, New Paltz. It can be used as an initial screening tool when Lyme and related diseases are suspected. Dr. Horowitz has found that a score of 46 or higher on the questionnaire implies a high probability of exposure to Lyme and other tick-borne illnesses.

What About Testing?

Laboratory testing for Lyme disease is problematic. This is partly due to the fact that the most common diagnostic tests for Lyme disease are indirect ones. They don't identify the bacteria itself, but instead look for antibodies to the bacteria. Unfortunately, for several reasons, someone with Lyme might not have measurable antibody levels. For example, the test may have been given too soon, before antibodies developed. Or, the immune system may be suppressed. Or, the person may be infected with a strain of the disease that the test can't detect. Thus, people who actually have Lyme may nonetheless test negative.

The two types of antibody tests that are most commonly used are the enzyme-linked immunosorbent assay (ELISA) and the Western blot. The ELISA measures the total amount of antibodies to *Borrelia burgdorferi* that are present in the blood. The Western blot identifies individual antibodies and looks for patterns that are unique to Borrelia. However, here's where things get complicated.

To understand why, it helps to know the difference between a "clinical" definition of Lyme disease and a "surveillance" definition. As Elizabeth Maloney, MD, explains in the Fall 2009 *Journal of American Physicians and Surgeons*:

Diagnostic criteria are situational. Clinical criteria are constructed to diagnose and treat ill patients. Research criteria are constructed to test a hypothesis in a uniform group of subjects...Surveillance criteria are much the same, the goal being selection of a homogeneous patient subset that can be observed over time and treatment.

At a public hearing in Connecticut in January 2004, CDC epidemiologist Dr. Paul Mead explained it like this:

Surveillance case definitions are created for the purpose of standardization, not patient care; they exist so that health officials can reasonably compare the number and distribution of "cases" over space and time. Whereas physicians appropriately err on the side of over-diagnosis, thereby assuring they don't miss a case. Surveillance case definitions appropriately err on the side of specificity, thereby assuring that they do not inadvertently capture illnesses due to other conditions.

Unfortunately, people with undiagnosed Lyme rarely find that their physicians "err on the side of over-diagnosis." Quite the contrary. Too often, the surveillance definition is misapplied in the clinical setting. Patients who initially test negative are simply told that they don't have Lyme disease, period. A more accurate and useful response would be, "Although you don't meet the CDC's strict standard for epidemiological surveillance, you may still have Lyme disease and there are other ways to figure that out." Instead, the opportunity for early treatment is lost.

According to Dr. Horowitz, the Western blot provides better information about the patient because it can detect antibodies specific to Lyme. He says that the presence of any Lyme-specific antibody strongly suggests exposure to the disease. Yet the Western blot has limitations as well. There are about 100 strains of Borrelia in the United States and about 300 strains worldwide. Some labs use multiple strains for testing, whereas, others use only one. Furthermore, some labs only look for certain bands (proteins) in the testing, while others look at all Borrelia-specific bands. In his book, Dr. Horowitz writes:

> *The utility of the Western blot is therefore based on the expertise of the laboratory performing the test, which strain(s) of Borrelia the patient was exposed to, and identifying the specific bands on the Western blot that reflect exposure to Borrelia.... We have found that a specialty lab, such as IGeneX, has a better chance of finding more Borrelia-specific bands on the Western blot, because it uses different strains of Borrelia burgdorferi for its testing.*

Like practically everything else related to Lyme disease, IGeneX's Western blot is considered controversial by some health care providers, due to the politics surrounding this disease. However, Dr. Horowitz states,

> *Lyme-literate doctors have used this laboratory effectively because it screens for more than just one strain of Borrelia. And every year IGeneX has passed stringent proficiency testing by the New York State Department of Health.*

Other Lyme tests include polymerase chain reaction (PCR), a DNA test, and a recently developed Lyme culture test by Advanced Laboratories. Moreover, there are a variety of tests for different co-infections, including antibody tests, PCR, and Fluorescent In-Situ Hybridization (FISH) tests. Dr. Horowitz also points out that there are different species of babesia, which require different tests.

> *If health care providers only check for Babesia microti, without checking for other strains like Babesia duncani (WA-1), and/or doing a Babesia panel with a PCR and FISH, they may miss the infection.... A negative Babesia test does not rule out the disease.*

Parents seeking to get to the bottom of their child's health problems often say to me, "What tests should I ask for? I'll have our pediatrician order them." Unfortunately, it's not that simple. These tests should not stand alone. Rather, they must be viewed as part of the overall clinical picture, and most importantly, the results should be read by a practitioner who knows how to interpret the findings.

PANS/PANDAS

Another condition can severely muddy the Lyme disease picture, complicating treatment and causing profound suffering. As with Lyme, it is poorly understood and fraught with controversy. It didn't even have a name until relatively recently.

In 1998, Dr. Susan Swedo of the National Institute of Mental Health reported on a devastating illness showing up in children. She called it Pediatric Autoimmune Neuropsychiatric Disorders Associated with Streptococcal Infections, or PANDAS. This bizarre constellation of symptoms starts with the sudden onset of obsessive-compulsive behaviors (OCD). At first, it was thought to be triggered by strep, hence the name. However, Dr. Swedo and colleagues came to recognize that Lyme disease and other infections can also cause this condition. In 2012, Dr. Swedo proposed re-labeling it Pediatric Acute-onset Neuropsychiatric Syndrome (PANS), to include cases not caused by strep. Since both terms are in general use, our book calls it PANS/PANDAS.

Dr. Charles Ray Jones summarizes symptoms and personality changes that PANS/PANDAS can bring on:

Symptoms:

Obsessions/compulsions

Motor and vocal tics

Choreiform movements (involuntary jerking or writhing)

Myoclonus (quick, involuntary muscle jerks)

Generalized anxiety (particularly bedtime fears)

Sudden personality changes may include:

Psychosis with hallucinations and delusions

Emotional lability (uncontrollable crying or laughing)

Oppositional defiance/rage

Separation anxiety

School phobias

Sensory processing issues

Issues with food (including anorexia)

Deterioration in cognitive functioning

Hyperactivity

Dr. Jones describes PANS/PANDAS as infection-induced autoimmune encephalopathy. In other words, it's what happens when an infection triggers an autoimmune response in the brain. He also calls it "brain on fire."

PANS/PANDAS is heartbreaking, frightening and profoundly disruptive to family life. Parents often say that they had no idea what was happening to their child. Some describe it as if their child's body was somehow taken over by an alien. Furthermore, they often find their physicians are as mystified by it as they are.

Lisa Kilion, mother of a child with Lyme and PANS, writes in her blog *PANS Life*:

> *Walk into a psychiatrist's office, and your child who unknowingly suffers from PANDAS or PANS is likely to be diagnosed with an onslaught of psych issues. You will be told she has anything from bipolar to OCD, from tic disorders to anxiety, from schizophrenia to borderline personality disorder. I'm not judging people who have these other diseases. But PANDAS is not a psychiatric disease, although it certainly presents as being just that.*

Kilion elaborates on some of the "shopping bag of symptoms" a parent might notice in a child with PANS/PANDAS. Among them:

- **Sensitivity to germs.** Exposure to colds, flu, or other infections may cause the child's symptoms to flare—bringing a resurgence of OCD, tics, depression, rage, body aches.

- **Changes in voice.** The child's once-sweet voice will now sound demonic and monotone. Or babyish. Or switch from one to the other. There may be stuttering.

- **Changes with eyes.** The child's pupils may dilate. Or a blank look, a faraway look, will emerge. Anger shows itself through the eyes, dark and flashing.

- **Pinocchio limbs.** Disjointed, flailing arms. Legs that don't want to hold up the body. It might seem like the child is faking it—falling to the floor, claiming she can't walk. But it's for real.

- **Rage and headaches.** Children with PANS/PANDAS may smash TV sets and computer screens or punch at doors.

Our appendix lists sources for more information about PANS/PANDAS.

four

Daily Life With Lyme Disease

Dorothy:

A LYME DIAGNOSIS for your suffering child often brings relief. Finally, some answers! Then, reality hits. Yes, there's now a path through the wilderness, but it's twisted and rocky, with unknown dangers lurking in shadows. How do you get through it?

In two-parent families, one parent (often the mother) may leave her job to care full time for the disabled child. Single parents don't usually have that option. They may have to patch together a solution with grandparents or other caregivers. Such changes may trigger resentment, anger, guilt, and anxiety in family members, including the child who is ill. It's complicated, but good organizational skills can help.

Medical Treatment

After the doctor has diagnosed your child with Lyme disease, it's time to start treatment. This usually involves antibiotics and/or other antimicrobial medications. The protocol might include herbal supplements to strengthen the immune system, and perhaps such adjunct therapies as chiropractic treatment or acupuncture. The physician may suggest dietary changes, such as eliminating sugar. Daily life is likely to change drastically.

Taking medications and supplements will become a ritual with almost religious significance. Antibiotics and other drugs must be taken at prescribed times of the day, either with food or on an empty stomach. Probiotics—to restore the "good" bacteria in the gut—need to be taken several hours away from antibiotics. Vitamins, minerals, and herbal supplements have their own timetables as well. With food or without, with other medications or several hours apart. It's essential to develop a system to keep track of all this. Your child's recovery depends on it. Ten years ago, my family kept a pill chart on a clipboard in the kitchen, next to the plastic tub full of medicines. Nowadays, there are pill tracker apps for your smartphone, such as Pillboxie and Pill Reminder, that can simplify the process.

You'll probably want a compartmentalized pill container, in which you count out a week's (or a month's) worth of pills at a time. As treatment continues and more medicines get added to the mix, you may need one with bigger compartments. A bead organizer from a craft store works nicely, offering more room than typical pill holders. It's also important to order drug refills before you run out. Sometimes the pharmacy is out of stock and needs to reorder. Or a special request needs to come from your doctor before the insurance company will pay for it. To avoid any lapses in medication, you need to build in some wiggle room.

Familiarize yourself with everything your child takes. Know what to look for in terms of possible side effects and potential interactions between different drugs. Your pharmacist, package inserts, and the National Institutes of Health's MedLinePlus website are good sources of information. Drugs.com also offers a free app that includes a drug-interaction tracker. If more than one practitioner prescribes for your child, let each of them know about all of your child's medications. Notify them of changes as they occur. Some physicians are set up to accept emails from patients. Otherwise, type up your new list of medications and supplements, and fax it to the doctor's office.

It is critical for parents to understand the Jarisch-Herxheimer reaction, often called "a herx." Herxing is a temporary flare of symptoms that sometimes—but not always—occurs during Lyme disease treatment. When the immune system is prodded by antibiotics to become more active, it releases inflammatory molecules called cytokines, which kill the bacteria. According to Dr. Horowitz,

> *These inflammatory molecules then create inflammatory symptoms, including increased fever, muscle and joint pain, headaches, cognitive impairment and a general worsening of the patient's underlying symptomatology. This is a major hidden reason why so many people with Lyme disease seem to get worse—and not better—when they are taking antibiotics.*

Herxes can indicate that the treatments are working, that the Lyme spirochetes are dying. However, sometimes the strong reaction will be very hard on the patient. Physical and behavioral symptoms can intensify dramatically. In children prone towards rages, herxing may trigger an increase in explosive behavior.

Discuss with your child's doctor the best way to manage herxes. Sometimes detoxification measures such as Epsom salt baths or herbal supplements can relieve discomfort. Other times, the doctor may decide to cut back or change the medication. Staying on top of herxes is essential during Lyme treatment. Furthermore, a worsening of symptoms doesn't always indicate herxing. It could be an allergy to the medicine or even something completely unrelated. It's important to alert the doctor whenever there is a significant change in symptoms.

Dietary Needs

Many Lyme-treating doctors say that improving diet is essential for recovery. Yet, dietary habits tend to be ingrained. Even healthy people may find it difficult to change what they eat. Modifying the diet of a sick child—and perhaps the whole family—can be a hard sell. However, recognizing how much it can help your child is a great motivator.

Anyone taking long-term antibiotics is typically advised to cut out sugar. This is to prevent yeast overgrowth, an uncomfortable and potentially dangerous condition called candidiasis. Most people have small amounts of candida organisms in their gastrointestinal tracts. These are normally kept in check by beneficial bacteria in the gut. However, as antibiotics kill off the "bad" pathogens, they also wipe out the "good" flora. This allows the yeast to run amok, which can result in problems involving the skin, genitals, throat, mouth, and blood. "Sugar feeds yeast directly," says Dr. Nicola McFadzean, author of *The Lyme Diet: Nutritional Strategies for Healing from Lyme Disease.* "Simple sugars are the easiest fuel source for it—so minimize the simple sugars in your diet to deprive Candida of its food source."

Lyme doctors also typically advise their patients to take probiotics. These microorganisms help replenish the gut with healthy flora. They are found in cultured and fermented foods, such as yogurt, kefir, sauerkraut, and miso. Be sure to look for "active and live cultures" on the label. Not everybody can tolerate fermented foods, however. Probiotics are also available in capsule and powdered forms. Most probiotic supplements need to be refrigerated to keep their potency. (There are a few exceptions.) Different brands of probiotics vary widely in quality. Ask your doctor which ones would be best for your child.

In her book, Dr. McFadzean examines what she calls the three pillars of Lyme treatment. They are:

1. killing pathogens;
2. strengthening the body (supporting the immune system, improving digestion);
3. reducing other stressors (heavy metal toxicity, hormone and other imbalances in the body, inadequate nutrition).

According to McFadzean, nutrition plays a central role in the second and third pillars. She writes: "Immune support, inflammation management, hormone regulation, and detoxification functions can all be vitally influenced by your nutritional intake."

A healthy diet of fruits, vegetables, and protein supplies the immune system with raw materials and also promotes healthy digestive function. Since 70 percent of the immune system resides in the gut, says McFadzean, it's important to maintain a healthy balance of intestinal flora. This avoids "leaky gut" syndrome, which can cause so many problems for Lyme patients.

McFadzean emphasizes the need to avoid gluten, a protein found in wheat, rye, and barley, which feeds inflammation in the body. People with Lyme already have inflammation triggered by the infection, she says. Thus, it makes sense to avoid eating anything that will add more fuel to the fire.

People have different levels of reaction to gluten. Those with celiac disease, an autoimmune disorder, must avoid it entirely, since eating any gluten at all can damage their small intestine and cause unpleasant symptoms. Others, including many with Lyme disease, may be sensitive to gluten, and feel better if they avoid it as well.

Removing gluten from your diet may seem hard at first. A good way to start is to focus on foods that are naturally gluten-free, such as fruits, vegetables, meat, fish, beans, legumes, nuts, and rice. Many people can't bear the thought of giving up bread, rolls, pizza crust, pancakes, noodles, and cookies. Luckily, gluten-free options for these have become more available in recent years. Although, unfortunately, such items usually contain sugar.

Canned and packaged foods, as well as meals prepared in restaurants, may have hidden gluten. For instance, you may not expect to find wheat in soy sauce, soups, or French fries, but it's often there. Read labels, and in restaurants, don't be afraid to ask how foods have been prepared. Another area of concern is prescription and over-the-counter medications. The filler that is added to the active ingredients often includes gluten. Frustratingly, manufacturers are not required to disclose this on the label. More information and support for going gluten-free is available on the website of the Celiac Disease Foundation.

You should also be alert to possible interactions between medications and food. For example, more than 85 different drugs should never be taken with grapefruit juice. Some medicines require avoiding dairy products. Mepron and Malarone, two drugs that treat babesiosis, must be taken with fatty foods for peak effectiveness. An online drug checker at healthline.com also lists interactions with food.

Your child may also have food allergies. According to FARE (Food Allergy Research and Education), a non-profit educational group, eight foods account for 90 percent of all food-allergic reactions in the United States. These are: peanuts, tree nuts, milk, egg, wheat, soy, fish, and shellfish. FARE's website gives useful information about living with food allergies. If you suspect your child has this kind of problem, ask your Lyme doctor about allergy testing.

About six months into Lyme treatment, my daughter suddenly developed allergies to almost anything she tried to eat. Even one bite of many different foods would make her throat start to close up and make it hard for her to breathe. At one point, her only "safe" foods were plain rice and a few kinds of fruit. Her doctor prescribed antihistamines and an inhaler, which made her less reactive. He also ordered allergy testing. Luckily, within a few weeks, the problem went away as quickly as it came on. We re-introduced foods slowly and found that she tolerated them well. I have heard reports of similar "temporary" allergies from other people with Lyme disease.

Figuring out what the child should or shouldn't eat is of course only part of the challenge. The bigger task can be to get the child and perhaps other family members to buy into the new dietary regimen. Sometimes there are hidden issues. One mother in my support group expressed her frustration with trying to get her 8-year-old son to eat gluten-free. She repeatedly told me, "He just won't stick to the plan." Yet, it turned out that there was a bigger problem. Her husband and older son persisted in bringing home many "forbidden" foods, which they would eat in front of the other boy. The sick child was supposed to be content with his carrot sticks and gluten-free crackers. Meanwhile his dad and brother wolfed down donuts and fudge brownies right next to him as they all watched TV.

I think these parents need to help both of their sons get some of what they want. For instance, maybe Dad could occasionally take the older boy out for something special—without rubbing his younger brother's nose in it. Healthy siblings deserve attention, too. On a different day, Dad might take the child with dietary restrictions out for gluten-free pizza. This way, each boy gets a treat and some one-on-one time with Dad, and nobody is made to feel bad about it.

Keeping Good Records

I used to say that the most important tools the parent of a chronically ill child needs are a three-ring binder and a three-hole punch. Now, I also recommend a smartphone and some apps. While the format may have changed over the years, you still need to organize a vast amount of information. You must monitor your child's symptoms, keep track of medications, and save a copy of every lab test and medical report. You need records of doctor appointments, prescriptions, and paperwork for filing insurance claims. It's a huge job.

Your smartphone can help you do this. Phone apps, like My Pain Diary and Symple, let you track symptoms and figure out connections. (Do certain foods seem to trigger headaches? After exercise, is it harder or easier for your child to fall asleep?) Apps let you record such information and then email PDF reports to yourself. You can either forward the email to the doctor or print out a hard copy and hand it to him in person. Since your child may go months between medical appointments, good records help the physician monitor your child's progress.

There are many apps that could prove valuable to a Lyme patient, and more are being developed all the time. "iMoodJournal" records moods and emotions. "Period tracker" helps your daughter stay on top of her menstrual cycle, when Lyme symptoms may worsen. "Paperless" and "Keep" offer easy ways to take notes and write checklists.

If you are comfortable using phone apps, they can help you maintain good records. But you can also use old-fashioned pen and paper. Some people jot symptom notes on a calendar and keep track of medications on a paper chart. The essential thing is to find a system that works for you—and keep at it.

You'll want to document every medical appointment, lab test, and procedure. Under federal law, you have the right to receive copies of your child's medical records, so be sure to ask for them. If test results are sent to you electronically, print out hard copies and put them in the binder, along with your other information. Bringing this file to your child's medical appointments will make office visits more productive. This way, you'll have all pertinent information at your fingertips, especially useful when seeing a specialist for the first time. (Note that your right of access does not extend to a mental health provider's psychotherapy notes. These are kept separate from the patient's medical records and are not available to you.) For more advice on keeping good records, see the book *My Lyme Guide,* by Marjorie Veiga and Dr. Sarah Fletcher. It contains practical forms and charts, along with explanations about how and why to use them.

It's also important to check with your accountant to see whether you meet the threshold for medical deductions on your taxes. For that, you'll need to document expenses, such as doctor visits, prescriptions, durable medical equipment, and medically related travel (including mileage, tolls, and parking fees). The cost of treatments, such as acupuncture, chiropractic care, and psychotherapy, are also deductible. For more information, see IRS Publication 502.

Modifying Your Living Quarters

If your child uses a wheelchair, you may need to modify your home. Major access problems, include entering and exiting the house, getting through internal doorways, and maneuvering within the bathroom. There are a variety of adaptive products. Portable wheelchair ramps, bedside commodes, and handheld showers can help.

Making major changes to the home can be a difficult decision for parents. It may be costly and disruptive to the whole family. Plus, there may be uncertainty about how long the changes will be needed.

For instance, when my daughter first started using a wheelchair, I couldn't imagine that she'd be in it for over three years. Parents may be understandably reluctant to remodel a house for what they assume is a temporary need. Furthermore, not all families are in a position to modify their living space, even if they want to. They may be renters and/or unable to afford such changes.

This is when it's important for family members to brainstorm creative solutions. If stairs are a problem, is there a first-floor room (or corner of a room) where the child could sleep? Can furniture be rearranged for easier access? Can snacks, remote controls, and personal supplies be kept where the child can reach them as needed? Although these changes might inconvenience parents or siblings, the rallying point must be that family members face their challenges together and do what's needed when one of them is ill. Looking at it this way may help take the pressure off of the child and reduce any guilt she may feel for bringing upheaval to the home.

A teenage boy with Lyme told me that most days he can get to his upstairs bedroom without too much difficulty. But sometimes, especially if he leaves the house with friends, his energy is sapped. By the time he returns home, he can't make it further than the living room and ends up sleeping on the couch. By allowing him this flexibility, the parents keep things as normal as possible. They support his need to socialize with friends, despite the price he pays in fatigue. The boy sleeps in his bedroom when he can, and makes other arrangements when he can't.

What Does Your Child Do All Day?

Children with Lyme tend to have problems with insomnia, fatigue, pain, and concentration. Some have daily fevers, vertigo, and other neurological problems. For many, this makes it impossible to attend school fulltime. Chapter Eight looks at educational options for children too sick to go to school. This chapter looks at the non-schooling aspects of a child's day. Obviously, variables of age, gender, health status, and temperament come into play.

No matter what else is going on, the medication schedule rules the day. You must get those meds into your child at the appropriate hour. If the child won't be home at pill time, meds need to be packed up and taken along. Also dominating the calendar will be medical appointments. Especially in the beginning, your weeks may be filled with doctors' appointments and lab tests. There may be alternative treatments, such as acupuncture, chiropractic, or hyperbaric oxygen therapy. All this can take an inordinate amount of time. Furthermore, patients often must go long distances to see their Lyme doctor. A LymeDisease.org survey published in *Health Policy* (June, 2011) found that most Lyme patients travel at least 50 miles for treatment. A sizeable minority travel more than 500 miles.

My family's case was typical. Our Lyme doctor was two hours away, and we also drove several hours per week to assorted therapies. Thus, we spent a lot of time in the car. Basic recommendations: Keep your vehicle gassed up. Know the good rest stops. And take appropriate snacks and entertainment options along with you. We discovered the locations of most of the Whole Foods Markets within a 100-mile radius of our house, which were good for gluten-free meals and wheelchair-accessible bathroom breaks. Now, there are also smartphone apps to help you find public restrooms as you travel, such as the "The Bathroom Map" and "Where to Wee."

A note about wheelchairs. Despite claims to the contrary, many businesses don't meet ADA guidelines for wheelchair accessibility. Barriers are everywhere. For instance, restaurants cram too many tables in a small space, stores put sales racks in the aisles, and trash cans may block the path to the restroom. One time Rachel and I were trapped inside the "accessible" dressing room of a discount store. Unbeknownst to us, a clerk had shoved a line of shopping carts against our door, so we couldn't open it. I'm glad my daughter wasn't in there alone.

"Good" Days And "Bad" Days

What does your child do when the two of you aren't burning up the freeway between home and the doctor's office? A lot can depend on whether it's a "good" day or a "bad" day. Good days may bring a burst of energy, a smile on your child's face and a flutter of hope in the parent's heart. Bad days can take different forms. Sometimes the child may have too much pain and fatigue to even get out of bed. There may be tears and despondency. Other times, the child may explode in anger and frustration. Besides being difficult to handle, this is incredibly demoralizing for the whole family.

A piece of advice from my co-author: "Don't ride the roller coaster." As much as possible, parents must stay calm, even as their child spirals out of control. I found this out first hand. If my daughter was very upset—angry or crying—any reaction from me could make things worse. Responding with anger or tears myself was like throwing gasoline on a fire. Seeming too pleasant or cheerful could backfire, too. She might think I didn't take her outburst seriously or didn't understand the extent of her pain and suffering. What worked best was to keep my expression neutral.

That is easier said than done, of course. All members of a household dealing with chronic illness are under immense stress, and sometimes they reach a breaking point. To mitigate that, I suggest using whatever resonates with you—prayer, deep breathing, silently counting to a hundred. Try your best to keep from feeding into your child's negative energy during the bad episodes. Hopefully, after the

66

storm passes, you'll be able to vent your own emotions outside the presence of your child, perhaps during a brisk walk around the block.

So, let's go back to those good days. Or at least the "less bad" ones. How does your child spend her time? Often, especially when the child is in a lot of pain, what's needed is distraction. Television, video games, audio books, music, and computers can help a lot. Books and magazines often don't work as well. Lyme can bring cognitive impairment, double vision, floaters, or other symptoms that make it difficult to read. Furthermore, children in pain need something to really pull their focus outside of themselves. For many, reading just doesn't do the job.

On the other hand, video games can capture a player's total attention, at least temporarily pushing away awareness of pain. Research studies have demonstrated the value of such games for pain relief. Experiment at home to find out which ones work best for your child. In addition to distraction, some games, such as "Wii Fit," have both physical and social components. If your child can stand up, he may benefit from some of the Wii's gentle balance activities. Since the games are fun to play, they are not only therapeutic for the child, but may be something the family can enjoy together.

TV programs and movies, if selected with care, can be real mood lighteners. A mother of a teenager with Lyme disease shared the following observations:

> *My 16-year-old daughter was always a straight "A" student—top of her class academically. Played AYSO soccer from a young age, volleyball in middle school then water polo her freshman year until she suddenly fell ill. She went undiagnosed for a year, in and out of three reputable hospitals and multiple doctors' offices. She was basically bedridden and we were doing a lot of crisis management due to cardiac and other autonomic complications.*

During this time she couldn't read due to encephalitis/headaches so we made a promise to only watch comedy shows and movies with happy endings. We upgraded to Direct TV with the ability to record. Every day we would scan the channels for uplifting entertainment and hit "record." The next day we would watch our happy selections and skip all the commercials. We watch "Ellen" and "Jimmy Fallon" daily together and laugh a lot. "The Voice," romance and Disney classics are always good too.

When my daughter first got sick, a neighbor lent our family a complete boxed set of the TV comedy *Friends*. We laughed our way through all 236 episodes, and then started over again from the beginning. We found out by personal experience what scientists have confirmed: there are physical benefits to sharing hearty laughter with others. According to research at Oxford University, watching 15 minutes of comedy along with other people increases one's tolerance for pain by 10 percent. It's not just distraction. The body's response to pain actually changes. It's important that it be a shared experience. Studies show that heavy laughter—the kind that produces an endorphin rush—is 30 times more likely to occur if you are with others than by yourself.

It's clear that TV, videos, and computer games can serve vital functions for the family dealing with chronic illness. However, in our case, it required a shift in maternal attitude. Before my daughter became ill, I had prided myself on how little television our family watched. And I was always horrified at the thought of letting children have a TV in their bedroom, with instant access, day or night. (I admit I was somewhat self-righteous about it.) Guess what? With a child homebound with Lyme disease, those standards flew out the window. TV and videos became our lifeline to sanity. Before we got Rachel's sleep problems under control, there were stretches when she was awake for 23 out of every 24 hours. We moved a TV into her room, with remote control and headphones, so that she could turn it on whenever she needed to. (This was before the days of streaming online videos. Today's options stretch far beyond the overnight infomercials for kitchen appliances and exercise equipment.)

Life Beyond TV and Videos

But what about experiencing life in ways that don't involve a TV or a computer screen? How can these young people learn other things, pursue hobbies that interest them, and see themselves as having a life beyond the confines of illness? That may sound like a tall order, especially when your household is in chaos. However, sometimes, it can be a path towards making things better.

Many young people enjoy music—listening to it, singing, and perhaps learning an instrument. One 17-year-old girl, who has had Lyme disease for years, has learned to play the bass guitar. She likes to play and sing along with recordings of different musicians. Reports her mother:

We once drove three hours round trip to see her favorite band perform. She loved singing along with someone whose lyrics have provided her such hope and encouragement. She said the singer's own struggles with illness have motivated her to persevere and to enjoy what health she does have. It gives me great joy to know that music helps my daughter cope.

More about the girl who only likes to watch movies with happy endings:

Now that she's in treatment we're having more good days. On days when her back isn't hurting she'll play the guitar or keyboard. She says it helps her get out of her head. She has a Pinterest where she gets creative ideas, then once a month we go to the craft store to get a project. She likes to paint bird houses, crochet & make bracelets.

She does Facebook to keep track of friends but sometimes it makes her sad when they're posting pictures of games or prom and all she has going on is physical therapy and doctor visits. She says her Tumbler gives her broader access to her favorite bands and what's happening in the world

One mother told me how her daughter has handled the cognitive impairments of Lyme disease.

She went from reading Jane Austen at age 12 to not being able to read simple sentences or do any math. Listening to the classics on audio books has been very helpful, along with Discovery Channel and Netflix for science-type stuff. When her hands can tolerate it, she will think of something to crochet and do it from her own mind. Patterns are incomprehensible right now.

She has a tablet now instead of a laptop, because the laptop was too heavy on her lap or to carry. She keeps up with friends on Facebook and plays Words with Friends with her grandma and some others.

Many children who are sick enjoy having pets. A teenager I know has cognitive impairment, which prevents many activities, but it doesn't stop her from training her dog. Feeding, brushing, and otherwise caring for pets can be gratifying to a child stuck at home. Yet, pets can bring problems to your family as well. For instance, indoor/ outdoor dogs and cats may carry ticks into the house, potentially exposing the whole family to a new batch of pathogens. Cats may be infected with a species of Bartonella that can be transmitted to humans by scratching. Reptiles may harbor Salmonella. Tropical birds can carry a number of diseases. If your family has pets, I urge you educate yourself about ways to diminish the health risks of pet ownership and consult your veterinarian for additional advice.

How can parents help children broaden their horizons? You start by supporting your child's interests, be it artwork, or Legos, or learning to knit. You help them find books, tapes, or movies that aren't just entertaining, but also include topics they care about. Some kids enjoy finding out—in small bites—about astronomy, life in the Middle Ages, or how ancient Egyptians built the pyramids. Parents should not "assign" such topics. That's too much like schoolwork. The key is to find things that capture the child's imagination. Learning that emerges from genuine interests can stimulate the child's brain without the pressure of school.

In my daughter's case, about a year into Lyme treatment, a present from her brother was a game-changer. After he bought himself a new computer, Jeremy gave Rachel his old one, which included Final Cut video editing software. Since at this point, she spent most waking hours in bed, we found an over-the-bed table to hold the computer. For hours a day, she taught herself to shoot and edit short movies, becoming quite accomplished at it. She could do it by herself or with others. She and a friend spent many hours figuring out how to do Claymation. They'd painstakingly craft little characters from clay, film them in different poses, and then edit it all together into an animated cartoon. It was creative, fun, and a bonding experience for the girls.

Developing a deep interest in something can help your child form relationships with other kids. A younger child might build things with K'nex or Legos, or make art projects with a friend who likes to do that, too. A teen might connect with others in person or via social media to share music or talk about movies. They might paint, or sew, or cook with friends. Strong interests make people more stimulating company for *themselves* as well as for others.

Journaling

The Diary of Anne Frank and *Zlata's Diary* are two internationally known journals written by girls living through horrendous circumstances. (The Holocaust and war in Bosnia, respectively.) These young authors recorded their experiences as they lived them, in a way that tangibly helped them in the moment. It happens that my daughter had read—and appreciated—both of those books in school, shortly before she got sick in seventh grade. Thus, early in her illness, when somebody suggested that Rachel start her own journal, it was not a foreign concept to her.

I was surprised at how readily she took to the idea, and how she kept at it for almost five years. Initially, she wrote by hand in a notebook. At some point, she switched to the computer. My husband and I never read it during the years she was writing it, honoring her request for privacy. But, I knew how important it was to her. She made time for it almost every day. When she wasn't writing, she'd often re-read entries from the past. When she shared it with us years later, I was struck by the range of emotions she expressed (and how good a writer she had become!)

Shari Brisson, coauthor of *Digging Deep: A Journal for Young People Facing Health Challenges*, knows what it's like to be young, sick, and scared for your life. At age 24, she was diagnosed with brain cancer and given six months to live. Writing about the topic in the North Dallas Gazette, Brisson states:

> *I can tell you, almost 30 years later that I'm still trying to get rid of that baggage. .... I honestly feel that if I had been better able to express my hopes and fears when I first had cancer, rather than trying to stay strong, I may have healed faster physically as well.*

Brisson calls journaling a simple, affordable, yet powerful, tool to help prevent emotional crises in young people with serious or long-term illnesses.

> *I don't mean a diary under lock and key to write about boy-crushes. I mean ...a journal to express ...how much it sucks to be in the hospital when their friends are all at homecoming. About how abandoned by their friends they feel. About how terrified they are they might die or never walk again or never have children! Kids with serious illness have these heavy, life-changing matters to get off their chests, and they have very little opportunity to do that without journaling.*

Each page of Brisson's book, *Digging Deep*, offers a writing prompt on a different topic, encouraging children to find new ways of looking at their situation. Some young people might do better with that kind of guidance. Others, like my daughter, started with a blank page or screen and did fine with it. I encourage you to experiment with your child and see if journaling is something he or she would like to try. For those who cannot write, due to their illness, voice-activated software may allow them to journal without actually typing on a keyboard.

What About Chores?

When Rachel was in the early days of her illness, before we knew she had Lyme disease, I read several books about chronic pain in children. What I still remember, ten years later, is how much those books emphasized having your child do chores. A prominent message seemed to be: don't let kids use their pain to escape responsibilities. Parents must firmly show these children they are expected to pull their weight around the house. Anything less would "send the wrong message." It would encourage laziness and teach the child to hide behind pain to get out of work.

This didn't sit well with me. These writers seemed oblivious to the reality of suffering children. At the time, my daughter was wracked with pain, 24/7. She couldn't stand or walk or sleep because of pain. Sometimes she had trouble breathing. These authors seemed to be saying that despite that, we should give Rachel a list of chores and insist that she do them every day. To me, the advice of these so-called experts made no sense.

Although I still disagree with those books about this, I now recognize something I didn't see before. It can be beneficial—even empowering—for a chronically ill child to participate in the everyday activities of the household. (I prefer not to say "chores," which implies drudgery.) Helping around the house may allow a child to feel more normal, more productive, and less of a burden. However, as with everything else, it depends on your circumstances.

In our experience, when Rachel's health was at its worst, she couldn't do anything. Many days she only left her bed to go to the bathroom. Trying to force her to do housework would have been heartless and ineffectual. However, with treatment, she reached a point where she was open to doing more. Although still in pain and often fatigued, she could manage "bite-sized" jobs, such as helping to set the table, peeling vegetables, or folding cloth napkins. We didn't force her do these things, and there was no penalty if she didn't feel up to it. Instead, we presented opportunities for her to help out in small ways, which didn't take long to complete but nevertheless made a contribution. This eased her transition from "bedridden patient" to participating member of the household. As her situation improved, she was able and willing to do more.

Social Life

A tough question that parents must grapple with is how to help mitigate their chronically ill child's isolation. There is no simple answer. Like everything else, it depends on the age of the child, how sick he or she is, what kind of social circle the youngster had before becoming ill, and what level of activity is possible now—among other factors.

Here are some general observations. A severely ill child might sometimes be unable to interact with anybody outside the immediate family. However, even very sick children may not be "out of it" all the time. Occasionally, they might feel well enough to yearn for the companionship of other kids. But that's not how childhood friendships tend to go. Children who are out of circulation for too long—not going to school, playing sports, or participating in other activities—may lose their connection to previous friends. Furthermore, other kids might feel uncomfortable around the sick child and prefer to avoid them.

I remember bleak stretches when my daughter was unable to leave the house and only rarely got out of bed. Friends called from time to time, but she was too impaired to see them or even talk on the phone. One by one, classmates and team members dropped away. Luckily, there were some neighborhood girls who stayed in touch through thick and thin. On days when Rachel was up to it, one or more of them would come over to watch videos, listen to music, or play a game. If she said she was too tired, they'd leave and come back another day. They were a lifeline for her, and frankly, for me, too. Their unwavering support helped her feel like her life included more than just four walls and a TV set.

Keep in mind that friends that come to visit don't have to be the same age. In fact, some experts believe that friendships between children of different ages can be very healthy for child development. Drawing on a large circle of potential visitors—cousins who live nearby, neighbors, peers that choose to stick around—broadens your child's pool of potential companions. When Rachel was bedridden at 14, an 8-year-old girl from down the street liked to come and paint pictures with her. Now, ten years later, they are still good friends.

If your child can leave the house, even occasionally, what social opportunities might there be? Perhaps you could bring a friend along when your family goes out to dinner or takes in a movie? What about youth activities at your place of worship? Keep it simple, being mindful of your child's energy level.

If your child is old enough, computers, tablets, and smartphones offer an opportunity to connect with friends via Facebook and other social media. They can also be used to play games remotely. While online games can be a fun way for homebound kids to stay in touch with others, these games can also be played with strangers, which we don't advise. It's important for parents to stay aware of their children's online activities and make sure they are making safe decisions. Common Sense Media is a website that provides parents with information and advice about media and technology. For example, here's what it says about the online game "Draw Something":

> Parents need to know that **Draw Something** is a takeoff of the popular **Pictionary** parlor game that's played with friends. While the game is fun to play with people you know, players can also compete with strangers online, which could expose them to inappropriate language and drawings. Learning to draw is fairly easy, which could make children want to play—but if they do so, it should be under strict supervision. The game also offers in-app purchases using real-world cash, but they are not essential. The free version of the app includes heavy advertising.

Other games, such as "Words with Friends" and "Trivia Crack" call for more skill. Many teens find those engaging. A bestselling game popular with all ages is "Heads Up," which combines aspects of a video game and playing with friends in the real world. It's an updated version of charades, available as a phone app developed by *The Ellen DeGeneres Show*.

Family Time, Holidays, Vacations

You certainly want your child's life to be about more than just being sick, and you want family life to be about more than that, as well. You want everyone in the family to feel that the child with Lyme disease is neither more nor less important than the others. Achieving this balance is a tall order. Brothers and sisters may find their own needs lost in the shuffle of medication schedules, doctor's appointments, and special diets. They may worry that their sibling will never get better, or that they will get sick themselves. They may feel guilty because their brother or sister is ill instead of them. They may resent having to assume more chores or seeing their home disrupted in order to accommodate their sibling. It's easy to imagine such scenarios when you are dealing with young children. You might assume it's not the case with brothers and sisters who are "old enough" to understand. Yet, that is not necessarily so.

My daughter's health problems started about the time my son left for college, making her an "only child" for the first time in her life. This simplified household logistics. However, Rachel's illness affected her brother in ways we didn't realize at the time. As I would learn years later, Jeremy worried very much about Rachel, his father, and me while he was away at school. He felt disconnected from what was happening at home and reluctant to burden us with anything going on in his own life. When he came home to visit, he found a changed world that revolved around the needs of his sister and felt excluded.

I have heard similar feedback from other families. In one case, a 22-year-old moved out and severed all family ties because of hard feelings about her younger sister's illness. Problems aren't limited to siblings, of course. Family stress takes a toll on spouses, as well. Sometimes marriages break up over it.

77

In an ideal world, parents would give each of their children and each other precisely the right amount and kind of attention. Every member of the family would pitch in as necessary to meet everybody's needs. But nobody lives in a perfect world, even without the challenges of illness. When chronic Lyme disease is part of the mix, family life can become truly chaotic. Parents must stay hypervigilant about their ailing child, whose needs may require immediate action. Some symptoms may even be life threatening, prompting visits to the emergency room. Along with medical issues, parents worry about other factors, too. Will he fall too far behind in school? Is she socially isolated? On top of it all, there may well be financial problems. Lyme disease treatment, often not covered by insurance, can deliver a knock-out punch to the family budget.

Engulfed in these overarching concerns, parents may be too overwhelmed to pay attention to how the family is functioning overall. Yet, it's important to step back, look at the whole picture, and decide how to keep things from getting too far out of control. (We discuss asking for help in Chapter 5.)

Despite these very real concerns, family life should be about more than just dealing with illness. It's important to find ways for the whole family to have fun together and nourish warm, supportive relationships among all of its members. Look for activities the whole family can take part in, such as board games or seasonal projects like carving pumpkins and decorating Christmas cookies. Card games like "Apples to Apples" can entertain all ages. If a child is too young— or cognitively impaired—to participate on his own, family members might play as teams. That would allow everybody to join in, perhaps sparing him the embarrassment of not being able to play well. Car rides can be enlivened with music or audio books that everyone can enjoy. Remember, anything you do—intentional or not—creates childhood memories. Let's strive to make them good ones.

For major holidays, think about what traditions your family already has, and look at ways to adapt them to your new situation. If you usually travel a great distance to stay with a houseful of relatives, maybe you'll choose to stay put and have a quieter holiday on your home turf. Perhaps some of those relatives would be willing to come to you—if that works for you and your family. It's important to celebrate the occasion in a way that is satisfying and fun for your family, rather than sacrificing your own needs to meet the demands or expectations of extended family members.

If you choose to travel, be realistic about what your family can reasonably handle. Sleeping in an unfamiliar bed and being removed from the comforts of home may take a huge toll on your child, which in turn will increase the stress on you. As ever, good planning is essential. You don't want to be miles away and realize that you left a medication at home. You may decide to use a pharmacy that's part of national chain so that, if necessary, you can refill prescriptions far from home. Be clear-eyed about your family's needs, and figure out how to meet them.

For the first two years that my daughter used a wheelchair, we didn't travel anywhere except to medical appointments. We celebrated holidays at home, and invited loved ones to visit when they could. Occasionally, Rachel would wistfully comment about how much fun it would be to go to the beach again, but that always seemed totally out of the question. Then, we found out about beach wheelchairs, which are specially outfitted with wide wheels that can go on sand and in the surf. It turns out that many beaches in California and other coastal states make them available for free or low-cost rental. We planned a trip to a beach near my son's college and made a family adventure out of it.

If you want to take a family vacation—and can afford one— think about ways to ensure success. For instance, even if your child doesn't normally need a wheelchair, you might use one for long treks through an airport to preserve his energy. Another item that can help a fatigue-prone child keep up is a portable motorized scooter. Available for rent in many vacation spots throughout the country, it can be folded up and carried in the trunk of a full-sized car. If staying in a motel, book a unit with a kitchen. This makes it easier to stick to dietary requirements and to refrigerate medications. Be realistic about your child's need for rest, and schedule appropriate breaks throughout the day.

Sensible planning can make the difference between triumph and failure. For costly vacations, consider trip insurance, in case your child is unable to travel at the last minute. Make sure you understand the limitations of the policy you purchase. "Cancel for any reason" insurance costs more, but may help avoid messy issues related to pre-existing medical conditions. See our appendix for travel-related resources.

Whether you are planning a vacation trip to the beach or just trying to keep your home life in some semblance of order, it's important to keep an open mind. Your child's situation is unique. Creative, out-of-the-box thinking can help parents find the best solutions for their family's needs.

Unique Challenges For Teenagers

Chronic illness poses special issues for teenagers. As one teen with Lyme wrote, "We depend on our parents so much for everything, yet we yearn for the independence that being sick doesn't bring."

While painfully aware that their peers are learning to drive, joining school clubs, applying to college, dating, and perhaps getting their first jobs, these adolescents are stuck at home, sick, and miserable.

The best advice I can offer here is to think in "baby steps." It's true that chronically ill teens can't be as independent as they'd like. Yet, it's important to figure out areas that they *can* control. Within reason, they should be free to choose how they spend their time and what energy they have. I've heard versions of the following complaint from more than one teen with Lyme:

> *Usually, I'm so wiped out that I can't do anything—not schoolwork, not talking to friends, certainly not leaving the house. Yet sometimes, I'll have a good day and get a little burst of energy. I want to go visit my friend but my mom always tells me I should catch up on my algebra.*

I've also heard the parents' side of the discussion. They usually respond like this:

> *She's so far behind in school! And most days, she's too fatigued to even look at her books. If she finally has a good spell, I think she should get cracking on her assignments.*

I recognize that parents are legitimately concerned about their teen's falling behind in school. However, in the big picture, a change of scenery and time spent with a friend will probably offer longer-lasting benefits than an extra session of math. Furthermore, social connections can help motivate young people to do what it takes to get well. This keeps them focused on taking their medications and going to doctor's appointments. If "having a good day" means being forced to do schoolwork, where's the incentive in that?

If your teen is in a wheelchair, issues related to independence are especially acute. My daughter chafed at the fact that she couldn't go anywhere without being driven by her dad or me in our van. Eventually, she and her neighborhood buddies came up with a different option. Her friends would take turns pushing her wheelchair to a restaurant a few blocks away from our home, so they could enjoy an outing without parental involvement. It was a small move toward independence that she really appreciated.

Another question is how to get your teen to "buy in" to taking responsibility for medications and supplements, following proper nutrition, and getting enough sleep? Like everything else, it depends very much on your circumstances. For instance, some young people with Lyme are too cognitively impaired to handle medications. But others can do it, with guidance. Once again, think of baby steps. Is there one small thing that your son or daughter can be in charge of? If and when that proves successful, can you add a second thing? And then a third? The idea is to slowly ramp up the level of responsibility. Teens with Lyme may face years of medical treatment. Being able to manage many of their own needs is an important step towards health and maturity.

However, I don't recommend that you turn over responsibility for psychiatric medications to your teen. The risk of dire consequences—either from honest mistakes or from an impulsive choice—is too great. For safety's sake, psych meds should remain under control of the parents.

I have heard mothers complain that their teens are in denial about having Lyme. These kids may resist taking medications and other parts of treatment, because they don't want to capitulate to the idea of being sick. If they are able to go out with friends, they may experiment with alcohol or engage in other risky behaviors. When you add the frustrations of being chronically ill to the impulsivity that can result from tick-borne diseases, you may be in a volatile situation. Family counseling may be called for here. (See Chapters Six and Seven.)

When More Than One Person in the Familly Has Lyme

When my daughter was at her sickest point, I thought life was hard. However, I realize now that my family was in a better situation than many. Only one of us had Lyme. With my son away at college and my husband employed, I could focus my energies on meeting Rachel's needs. Later, when I became involved in Lyme advocacy work, I came to recognize that many people face more difficult and complicated circumstances. Sometimes several family members have Lyme. Sometimes the whole family is ill.

This can cause extreme hardship on many levels. The family's main wage earner may be out of commission. The cost of Lyme treatment is multiplied several times over. Ailing adults may barely be able to care for themselves, let alone their children. Sick kids who need nurturing may find it in short supply.

In one family I know, both parents and all four children were eventually diagnosed with Lyme disease. But it didn't happen all at once. Their oldest son was bitten by a tick at age 7, and subsequently began to suffer many different symptoms that no one suspected might be Lyme-related. His teenage years were punctuated by psychiatric issues and physical illness. At age 21, he was finally diagnosed with Lyme and began treatment.

His Lyme doctor noticed that other family members exhibited suspicious symptoms, though not as overwhelming as the oldest boy's. At the physician's suggestion, all were evaluated and found to have Lyme. Looking back now, the mother says she had felt poorly for years. Yet she had always assumed the headaches, fatigue, insomnia, and pain were brought on by the stress of dealing with her son's difficult adolescence. With Lyme treatment, her symptoms resolved, returning her to a level of mental clarity and physical stamina that she had thought she'd never see again.

Sometimes multiple family members have Lyme because they spend time in the same tick-endemic areas. Other times, it's because the mother has undiagnosed Lyme and unwittingly passes it to her children during pregnancy. Complicating the picture, children harboring the infection don't necessarily show it right away. They may fall ill at different times, with different symptoms. One may have problems paying attention in school, while another develops crippling pain in his legs.

Even if they begin treatment together, family members may not recover at the same time. Some may improve substantially and move on with their lives, while a sibling or parent does not. Such disparities can add to the family's heartache. I know one mother whose two sons were both bedridden from Lyme disease as young teenagers. For several years, both were treated by the same doctor. One boy improved enough to attend an out-of-state university, earn his degree, and start a career. Yet, his brother remains ill. He lives at home, continues treatment, and can manage only an occasional class at a local community college.

A mother whose family had Lyme says that her teens had to "accept their illness in order to get past it." They had to assume responsibility for taking their own medicine, eating a proper diet, and getting adequate rest.

Since I was unwell myself, I couldn't do everything for them. We helped each other along as best we could, but each one had to handle their own primary needs... Probably the most beneficial thing we did in the long run was to a see a family counselor. I had to learn how to set boundaries with my sick children. I had to decide how much to help them, and how much to let them learn to rely on themselves.

This mother said a positive thing that came out of this experience was the fact that family members really bonded with each other through their shared ordeal. "We learned to take care of ourselves and each other," she said. "We learned to be grateful for what we had. And we learned to have compassion for people going through hard times."

five

The Vital Importance
Of Boundaries

Sandy:

PERSONAL BOUNDARIES are limits set by individuals to protect and maintain healthy relationships with others. They define each person's right to self-determination and respect. For example, children learn boundaries when they are permitted to close the door when they're using the bathroom, and the adults respect the limit the child has set. There are areas, of course, in which parents must make decisions for the health and well-being of the child. However, whenever parents can respect the child's boundaries, it helps the child learn the importance of boundaries in their own lives, knowledge that they will carry with them even into adulthood.

Boundaries don't have to be static. They can change within relationships, depending on circumstances. Consider the following examples:

- A parent might not allow a 2-year-old to close the door when using the bathroom, needing to monitor the child.

86

But that same parent might allow a 3-year-old to close the door, once the child has demonstrated an ability to handle this situation.

- A healthy 12-year-old may be allowed to play ball down the street with friends. However, a child with sudden-onset rages from tick-borne illness may need constant adult supervision.

- The mother of a child with Lyme has always felt free to discuss anything with her sister. But then her sister doesn't accept that the child is really sick. She second-guesses the mother's decisions regarding diagnosis, treatment, discipline, and school issues. In that case, the mother needs strong boundaries with her sister, to protect herself, her child, and her family.

Adults respect boundaries when they recognize that other adults have the right to make decisions about their own lives. For instance, adult children don't necessarily check with their parents when they are mulling over major life decisions—marriage, divorce, or a move to a foreign country. They might ask their parents' opinion about the matter, or they might tell them about it after the decision has been made. In healthy adult relationships, both parties accept that people have the right to define and maintain their own boundaries.

Unfortunately, where Lyme disease is concerned, boundaries are often blurred. Relatives and friends may interfere, challenging the parents' decisions regarding medical treatment, education, and even child rearing. The family is already vulnerable, with their lives turned upside down by their child's catastrophic illness. Without appropriate boundaries, the fragile structure that the parents have built can crumble. Strong boundaries bring clarity. They create an atmosphere in which the parents and child can develop confidence in their decision-making and move forward in life. Let's look at one example:

Grandma arrives in town for a two-week stay. Since she lives far away, she doesn't visit often. She and her kids and grandkids love the time they spend together. Particularly eager to see her grandchildren, she focuses her attention on them. She joins them in playing with Legos, dolls, and stuffed animals, and they teach her how to play their electronic games. They have wonderful meals together. Grandma tells stories about her life in Chicago, and her children and grandchildren talk about everything they are doing in Virginia. The distance of time and place seems to fade away, as they easily reconnect with one another.

This trip, however, takes a very different turn. It's the first time Grandma has seen 8-year-old Charlie since he was diagnosed with Lyme disease. Over the phone, it had sounded quite serious. But now, seeing him in person, Grandma thinks Charlie looks fine, if a little quieter than usual. She wonders why he isn't in school, and why he doesn't have homework or assigned chores. It disturbs her to see Charlie picking at his food and staying up so late at night.

At first, Grandma had believed what her daughter Heather had said about Charlie's illness and the family's search for answers. But, now that she's seen the situation with her own eyes, she believes that things don't add up. She questions whether her grandson is feigning symptoms to get more attention or to avoid going to school. Why do his parents let him stay up all hours of the night watching TV? Why can he skip family meals and eat whenever he feels like it? She thinks this 8-year-old boy is playing his parents for fools and can't understand why Heather allows this.

By day three, Grandma has had enough. She tells her daughter precisely what she thinks about the whole situation. First, she says,

Heather needs to take Charlie for a second opinion. In fact, her neighbor's son is an infectious disease specialist at a major medical center nearby. They could go there. She has already called her neighbor and told her about what is going on. Her neighbor contacted her son, who said that Lyme disease is overdiagnosed and easily treated with two weeks of antibiotics. If it takes longer than that to treat, it's not Lyme. He would know. He is, after all, an important doctor. Grandma tells Heather to stop listening to that quack she is taking Charlie to.

Furthermore, Grandma says, stop babying the boy! Charlie should eat with the family—or go without meals. He should be in bed by 8:30, with lights out and no TV. As for school, he should go every day and do all of his homework, or else lose privileges. On a roll now, Grandma says, "Heather, I raised you to know the value of structure and discipline. I'm disappointed to see you let Charlie run roughshod over the family. He has to learn that such behavior won't be tolerated. And as for me, I'll play with my other two grandchildren, but I won't spend any time with Charlie until he shapes up. And I'll tell him that to his face."

Grandma has veered into what is clearly not her business. Let's look at some of the ways Grandma has crossed boundaries with Heather's family:

- She assumes that because Charlie doesn't look sick, he is not ill—and blames the parents for treating him as though he is.
- She assumes that her daughter and son-in-law aren't capable of making good choices for their family and attacks their decisions.
- She has betrayed Heather and her family by talking to others about their private business.

- She announces that she will not interact with Charlie unless he changes, thus punishing him and giving preferential treatment to his brother and sister.

Grandma needs to take a step back. It is not her place to make medical decisions for Charlie. She should not judge her daughter and son-in-law for how they are handling the situation. However, as a loving grandmother, it *is* within her role to talk privately with Heather. Respectfully, she can share her observations about Charlie's situation and ask for more information. She also needs to understand that her daughter can decline to engage in that conversation. Respecting boundaries includes accepting the other person's right to say "no."

If she can do this, and if Heather is willing, Grandma will discover much about what is going on in her daughter's family. She'll hear about their struggles with a child who is very limited physically, due to an illness that is controversial in the medical world. She'll learn that Charlie has an invisible illness and that looks can be deceiving. She'll find out that Charlie suffers from insomnia. He almost never gets restorative sleep—the deep, restful sleep that helps replenish the immune system. Non-restorative sleep is a common symptom of Lyme disease in children. Heather will explain how Charlie's blurred and double vision makes it hard for him to read, and about his food sensitivities and gastrointestinal problems, so typical of children with Lyme disease. She'll learn how isolated and attacked Heather feels when those around her make judgments based on how Charlie looks. If Grandma is open to this conversation, she can become a source of support and encouragement for her daughter, instead of just one more person who doesn't understand.

But, what if Grandma won't do this? What if she refuses to set aside her own assumptions, in order to learn about the needs of her grandson and his parents? What should Heather do then?

Boundaries are the guardian of oneself, the protector of one's personhood. Being aware of boundaries and enforcing them also protects our relationship with others. Let's look at what that means. In all of our relationships, we need to develop a sense of when something is or is not our business. Many of us were raised with hazy boundaries. We didn't respect other people's choices when they differed from our own. Maybe we thought everyone should eat the same things that we ate and vote for our same political party. Maybe we looked down on people who dyed their hair purple or pierced their noses. Some of us grew up believing that our religion, or lack of one, was superior to the beliefs of others. Or that our neighborhood or part of the country was better than other places. All of this can be a set up for problems with boundaries.

Boundaries require us to be open to the fact that other people are entitled to make their own choices in life. These might not be the same ones we would make, and they might even turn out badly. But the chooser has the right to decide and will live with the consequences.

Now let's go back to Charlie's story. He had been ill for about two years at the time of Grandma's visit. For months, his parents had watched his health decline, as they went from doctor to doctor seeking answers. Charlie suffered daily headaches that no medication could alleviate. He was highly sensitive to light and sound. At holiday time, the noise and lights of a shopping mall would trigger a severe migraine headache. He had trouble sleeping through the night. It was hard for him to read or do math. Yet, to those who didn't know better, he appeared perfectly normal. Unfortunately, the fact that he looked healthy affected how he was treated by extended family, neighbors, friends, teachers, and most health care professionals. Many didn't believe that he was sick and had very little patience with him, perhaps judging him as malingering, lazy, manipulative, or selfish.

Six months prior to Grandma's visit, Charlie's parents had finally found a specialist who figured out what was causing their son's many symptoms. The doctor diagnosed Charlie with Lyme disease and co-infections, and prescribed antibiotic treatment. The physician, who had treated thousands of children with chronic Lyme, told the parents that it might take many months to see improvement. In fact, the doctor warned them, Charlie's symptoms might flare from time to time, making it even harder for him to function.

In the above example, we see how Grandma's failure to respect boundaries affected her relationship with her children and grandchildren. Now, let's look at the scenario from her daughter's point of view.

Heather has always trusted her mother's judgment, and the two have always had a warm loving relationship. Now, the daughter feels both wounded and confused by her mother's attack. She begins to second-guess the decisions that she and her husband have made. Should they stop the medication? Should they go to yet another doctor? Should they force Charlie to go to bed even when he can't sleep? Heather and her husband had talked long and hard about how to handle their son's illness and had come up with a game plan that worked for their family. Changing it now, just because Grandma said so, might anger her husband and upset Charlie. But, after these strong objections from Heather's mother, some doubts are creeping in.

Grandma's visit, once so happily anticipated, has undermined the delicate balance this family had achieved. How will Charlie react to Grandma's hostile treatment towards him? Will his siblings turn on him as well, following Grandma's lead? Will Heather and her husband lose faith in their doctor and decide to stop treatment? Unless Heather can set and maintain boundaries with her mother, the damage to her family could be significant.

Chronic illness in a child can be emotionally overwhelming for a family. What may at first seem like an ocean wave can quickly become a tsunami. When extended family members overstep their boundaries and start telling the parents what to do, things can become even worse. It is the job of grandparents, aunts, uncles, and family friends to pay close attention to boundaries. There can be a delicate line between providing support and interfering. Maintaining clear boundaries helps to clarify everyone's roles. Not only does the child feel safe and protected, but the parents do, as well.

Shelly first came to see me about two years ago, at age 12, when she had been struggling with Lyme disease for about a year. She was unable to attend school, due to profound fatigue, sensory issues, and headaches. On some days, she couldn't even get out of bed. Shelly's mom and dad work full time and have two younger children. As they cared for Shelly and addressed her many needs, they also tried to keep things normal for her siblings, with both school and after-school activities.

Occasionally, Shelly's Grandma would come with her and her mother for our sessions. Since Mom and Dad did not want to leave Shelly alone in an empty house while they went to work, Grandma and Grandpa had volunteered to care for her on some days. Shelly enjoyed spending time with her grandparents. Both retired, they provided her with lots of time and attention. They gave her medications, prepared foods for her special diet, and kept her company. Grandpa and Shelly often watched programs together on Animal Planet and the History Channel. Grandma and Shelly would do arts and crafts on days when Shelly wasn't too fatigued.

Shelly may have been infected eight to ten years before being diagnosed with Lyme and starting treatment. Her symptoms were largely neuropsychiatric, including severe problems with cognition and executive functioning. She couldn't even follow simple directions and struggled with homebound instruction. When I first met Shelly, I was astonished by the level of support she and her parents received from her grandparents. Although Shelly was quiet during most of the session, Grandma watched the girl's facial expressions closely. She could tell when her granddaughter was becoming upset, even when Shelly couldn't express it. Grandma would gently ask Shelly to let me know what was bothering her and helped her find the words.

To my knowledge, Grandma and Grandpa never doubted Shelly or her parents. They provided support with no strings attached— no judgments, no attacks, and no manipulation. How wonderful for Shelly and her parents to have Grandma and Grandpa in their camp! The family was stressed over Shelly's medical care, battles with their insurance company, and the need to advocate with the school. But they didn't have to worry about Grandma and Grandpa, a quiet constant in their lives. This was a profound gift from the grandparents to Shelly and her family, without fanfare. They were just present.

I started with grandparents because they can be either a major support or an obstruction. When they or anyone else crosses boundaries, parents need to recognize it and immediately set limits. It is always disrespectful to cross boundaries. It is not at all disrespectful to identify when boundaries have been crossed and take appropriate control. For instance, going back to Heather, she might say, "Mom, we love to have you visit. But, we won't invite you back if you don't respect our decisions and our right to make them. We want you to be part of our lives, treating us all fairly and not judging us or interfering with how our family works. If you want to know more about Charlie's illness, I'd be happy to discuss it with you. But only if you are seeking to understand and not to judge or second-guess us." When there is a history of a respectful relationship, attending to boundaries can restore that respect, getting everything running smoothly again.

However, when that history of respect in the relationship doesn't exist, other strategies are needed. Sometimes extended family members don't respect boundaries at all. They believe that by virtue of being the child's grandmother, aunt, or uncle, they are entitled to say and do whatever they like. In those cases, some families may find it necessary to cut off contact, or restrict it to telephone calls and e-mails. I believe that families with chronic Lyme disease should not compromise on boundaries. There is too much at stake. The parents and child must feel safe and protected, in order to navigate the complex problems that this illness produces.

For many families, dealing with other people's responses to their chronically ill child can be very complicated. Some boundaries are not obvious and may be unique to children with Lyme. For example, extended family members may reach out to hug the child when they visit. If she has severe body pain or is especially sensitive to touch, she may not want to be hugged. A visit will generally go better if the parents let others know this in advance. By clarifying for guests what behavior is and is not acceptable, parents protect their child from the very start of the visit. It also protects the relationship between the guest and the child.

Here's another boundary: guests should not comment on the child's functional problems—such as whether a child stays in bed for a long period of time with the shades closed tightly. Again, visitors should be told what to expect beforehand and asked not to mention any of it.

Then there is food. Children with Lyme may have dietary restrictions or aversions to some foods (often part of their sensory sensitivity issues). In that case, parents should ask guests not to bring food and not to talk about changes to the child or family's eating habits. These practices may seem odd to those who don't have Lyme, especially grandparents who love bringing candy and other desserts. When setting this boundary, parents could suggest non-edible gifts, such as a game or Lego kit.

Aunt Bonnie might be crushed that she can't bring her famous pumpkin pie for Thanksgiving dinner. But Aunt Bonnie needs to realize that the focus should be on the sick child's needs and not her own feelings. Bringing Lego kits to dinner instead of pie supports the family and respects their boundaries. (Of course, Aunt Bonnie could also consult with the parents and find out if her pie recipe can be adapted to meet their dietary needs. Gluten-free crust, perhaps? Maybe using stevia as a sweetener, instead of sugar?)

Loving visitors who don't see a child regularly may notice that she looks healthier than she had in the past. It would be natural for them to say, "Jane, I'm glad to see that you're getting better." For some children with Lyme, however, this is not a welcome comment. They don't see it as a supportive remark, but rather as a denial of their illness and their pain. If you think your child might react that way, warn visitors not to comment on any sign that the child is recovering. Most children with Lyme do best when people around them acknowledge and validate their illness, yet spend time with them in cheerful ways.

Here's what they might say instead: "Jane, it's great to see you! Would it be all right if I give you a hug?" Or, "Jane, I see that you're in bed today. Do you want some company? If you would like, we could watch a movie together, or I could read to you." Giving choices to a child respects her boundaries and improves the relationship. Sick children can feel very isolated. It is a gift to have a trustworthy loved one spend time with the child. This expands her limited world and takes some pressure off of the parents. A visitor who respects boundaries can help cut through the isolation.

Knowing how to set and maintain boundaries can be vital for parents. Overwhelmed by caring for a sick child, trying to keep the family afloat, and figuring out how to pay the high costs of treatment, parents might initially be inclined to overlook the boundary issues and just let things go. However, parents can pay an enormous price for that. On a concrete level, interfering relatives and friends could compromise the child's treatment. For example, they might convince the child that she "doesn't really have Lyme disease." Therefore, she may refuse to take her medicine or stay on her diet.

There are tangible benefits when parents push back against those who cross boundaries. For many parents of children with Lyme, months or years of misdiagnoses and ineffective treatment have eroded confidence in their own judgment. Once they finally receive a Lyme diagnosis, they see that they were not wrong to keep digging and leave "no stone unturned." Hope that their child can get well returns and, along with it, some much-needed self-assurance.

Yet, when other parties intrude on the family's boundaries, it wears away at that confidence. This makes it harder for the parents to navigate their complicated situation. Conversely, identifying boundaries and keeping them intact protects the family. Strong boundaries shore them up and increase their confidence to make and alter daily decisions, as needed.

Is there a respectful way for others to provide input to the parents, without crossing boundaries? As a psychotherapist, a mother, grandmother, and Lyme patient, I most assuredly say "yes."

In our initial example, Grandma may request a time to talk privately with her daughter and son-in-law. She can ask if they are open to questions. (Grandma must be willing to accept any answer—yes, no, or not now). Admitting her own lack of knowledge of the disease can be helpful. ("You and your brother never had trouble sleeping, so this surprises me. Why is sleep such a problem with Lyme?") Here, Grandma seeks information in a non-accusatory way. Openness is essential, if others want to be close to the ill child and family. Learning about the illness and her grandson's struggles will help Grandma find ways to support Charlie, Heather, and the whole family.

Boundaries are not just for family and friends. Parents may also have to set limits with doctors or school officials. Once there is a diagnosis of Lyme, parents may decide against taking their child to any medical practitioner who denies chronic Lyme. However, even when under the care of a Lyme specialist, their child still needs a primary care doctor. Not wanting to undermine the child's treatment, the family may look for a doctor who is open to the Lyme diagnosis. If there are specialists involved (neurologist, cardiologist), parents may seek out those who are not hostile to Lyme, if they are available. To provide for the emotional safety of their child and their family, they need to assemble a team they can trust.

Boundaries regarding school are also important. For instance, if the child is on homebound instruction, do the tutors recognize the child's cognitive issues? Do they understand how symptoms such as headaches and profound fatigue make it difficult for the child to do assignments? Do they respect the child's need for breaks? (For more about boundaries with schools, see Chapter Nine.)

Setting and maintaining boundaries can be complicated, particularly for parents who have never found the need to look at these issues in the past. As parents go through this process, it is important to *respond* rather than *react* to situations that arise. Unless there is a critical need to act quickly, I tell parents to pause, think about the situation, and plan their next steps, rather than acting on impulse. Ideally, with both mother and father on the same page, parents would have a unified approach to any situation that arises. Many clients have told me that learning about boundaries has been incredibly helpful to them, offering a life-changing approach to all of their relationships.

Dorothy:

We learned about the importance of firm boundaries during the years my daughter was in the wheelchair. And the boundary-crossers weren't always people we knew. Sometimes, they were total strangers. I discovered that many adults thought nothing of going right up to my wheelchair-bound daughter and asking, "What's wrong with you?" How is a young teenager—or anyone—supposed to answer that? (It would seem ill-mannered to say "mind your own business," although that's what we both wanted to tell them.)

This was particularly distressing early in Rachel's illness, when we didn't *know* what was wrong. If she truthfully answered "I don't know," it only prompted more questions. "What do you mean you don't know? Did you hurt yourself? Are you sick?" Rachel and I came to dread meeting people who felt free to say and do whatever they liked.

We were astonished by how many people tried to give her a "friendly" touch on her shoulders, not knowing how painful that would be for her. At age 15, Rachel wrote about this in an essay published in *The Lyme Times*.

> *Because I just look like a regular girl sitting in a wheelchair, adults always seem to want to pat me on the shoulder—even people I've never met before. When people approach me, I have to remember to turn my wheelchair to block them from touching my shoulders. Many people don't pay attention to that signal, reach over and pat me anyway. My friends and I joke about putting spikes on my shirt, but I doubt that would help.*

Inappropriate behavior on the part of adults (not respecting her personal space or her privacy) happened over and over again. Apparently, many adults assume they are entitled to ask a child anything. Once, a teacher from a different class came up to Rachel at school and said, "Tell me everything that has happened to you, starting from the beginning." This woman probably thought she was being sympathetic and supportive. In fact, she put my daughter in an uncomfortable spot. Rachel had no desire to share such information, but it would be considered rude for a student to say that to a teacher. This adult did not respect boundaries. Luckily, the teacher was called away before the conversation went further.

Rachel and I devised strategies for protecting her from such unwelcome incursions. Our game plan was for her to say something vague and then quickly change the subject. For example, if somebody asked her why she was in the wheelchair, she might respond, "Oh, I've got some health problems... (turning head and pointing)... Hey, look at that butterfly!"

Recently, the mother of a teenager with Lyme emailed me for advice about a similar situation. Reeling from her daughter's grueling illness, she felt bombarded by questions from all sides. "People keep demanding answers, and I don't know what to say."

I told her what I told Rachel so many years ago. Just because somebody asks a question, doesn't mean you have to answer it. *You* decide what, if anything, to tell them. This is part of maintaining good boundaries. Answer the questions you want to and then change the subject. ("Did you catch the latest episode of Downton Abbey last night?")

Of course, there are people in your life to whom you want to explain more. Even so, it should be on your own terms. You decide how much mental and emotional energy to spend. Sometimes, the answer may have to be, "I'd be happy to give you more details, but can't today. I'm too tired." When the situation with my daughter was at one of its lowest points, I was grateful for how one of my friends responded. She said, "I'm interested in whatever you want to say. But you don't have to tell me anything. We can talk about other things or be silent if you like." That was a gift.

Asking For Help

Enforcing boundaries doesn't mean that you can't ask for help from the people in your life. In fact, clear boundaries allow you to define what kind of help you need and how best to receive it. Toni Bernhard, author of *How to Be Sick: A Buddhist-Inspired Guide for the Chronically Ill and their Caregivers*, asks in her blog:

> *How many times have you said to a friend or relative in need, "Let me know if there's anything I can do to help," and when you didn't hear back, failed to follow-up? I've lost count of the number of times I did just that—failed to follow-up when I didn't hear back from someone in need, even though I would have been happy to help in any way I could.*

According to Bernhard, the person who needs the help must specify what assistance is needed and on what terms. This is an extension of the concept of boundaries.

Make a list of supportive friends or extended family that could step in and assist you. Figure out what kind of help could keep your household running smoothly and provide a sense of stability to the family. Shopping? Cooking? Shuttling siblings to music lessons or soccer practice? Some families use websites like Lotsa Helping Hands or Caring Bridge to organize this kind of assistance. It can be trickier to get someone to take over direct care of the sick child. If that can be arranged, however, it can give parents a welcome break. Yet, even the most caring of friends and family must observe appropriate boundaries. This can be helped by being very specific in your requests: "Are you available to take Patrice to her piano lesson at 3 p.m. on Friday?" "Can you deliver my car to the repair shop at 9 a.m. on Tuesday?"

Sometimes families are in the uncomfortable position of having to ask others for financial help. For many people, this is very difficult. If you find yourself in that situation, I suggest you make your request in private. Let the person know how sick your child is, how difficult it is to find care, and then state your case simply and forthrightly. "This treatment is going to cost $10,000, and we have no way to pay for that right now. Would you be able to lend us the money?" Recognize that this is also a boundaries issue. The person you are asking has the right to say no. However, many families struggling with Lyme disease find that grandparents and other relatives are willing to provide financial help when they realize that the need is great.

six

The Role Of Psychotherapy
And Family Therapy

Sandy:

FOR SOME PARENTS AND CHILDREN confronting the challenges of Lyme disease, psychotherapy, or family therapy can be a big help. Before seeking a psychotherapist, however, there are a number of things to consider. Different therapists use a wide variety of techniques in their work with clients. Methods that work well for the general client population may not be effective for Lyme patients. Some may actually be counterproductive.

For example, if the therapist doesn't realize that fatigue in Lyme patients is far beyond merely being tired, she may expect more than the patient is capable of doing. If she doesn't understand the reason for long-term medical treatment, and the adolescent complains about being on antibiotics, she might support the girl's position, and encourage her to stand up to her parents on the issue. Without knowing the complexities of tick-borne diseases, a therapist may not understand the many reasons why patients cannot attend school for long periods of time, or go away to college right after high school graduation.

One goal of psychotherapy is to promote improvements in the way a client functions—going to school or work, doing well there, being able to do errands and chores. Yet, for many Lyme patients, no amount of psychotherapy will improve their ability to function. That's because their functional problems stem from their physical illness, which won't be fixed without effective medical treatment. A therapist who knows this will understand the need to help the Lyme patient set different goals than could be reachable for a client that does not have Lyme.

There is widespread misunderstanding of Lyme disease in the medical arena. Just reaching a diagnosis of Lyme disease can be a traumatic experience for the child and the whole family. This trauma, on top of that caused by the illness itself, can give rise to issues not present among others seeking therapy, even those with most serious illnesses.

Consider the following scenario, one I commonly see with families in my practice. When their child first starts exhibiting joint pain, headaches or other symptoms, the parents take her to the pediatrician. Not recognizing that she may have Lyme disease, he tries a variety of treatments that do not bring relief. Then he refers them to a rheumatologist or other specialist, who also fails to consider that Lyme disease might be the cause of this child's illness. He tries a variety of treatments that don't help either. The child continues to complain about pain and misses a lot of school because of it. Suspecting that the problem is psychosomatic, the doctors give up exploring underlying medical explanations. They refer the child to a psychiatrist.

The psychiatrist, who also doesn't know much about Lyme disease, presumes that these symptoms are caused by a mental illness and prescribes psychiatric medication. With undiagnosed Lyme disease, those drugs may have a paradoxical effect or none at all. Then, the psychiatrist becomes convinced that the child is mentally ill. He may even decide it's severe enough for her to be admitted to a psychiatric hospital. In the hospital, this child with undiagnosed Lyme disease will be "treated," perhaps with more psychotropic medications, along with individual and group therapy. All of this treatment is focused on the psychiatric illness that the doctors have presumed this child certainly has.

In my experience, many Lyme patients are misdiagnosed with mental illness because doctors fail to uncover the physical origin of their symptoms. The problem is not limited to tick-borne diseases. According to Harvard psychiatrist Barbara Schildkrout, more than 100 physical ailments can manifest symptoms that appear to be mental illness. In her book *Unmasking Psychological Symptoms*, Schildkrout writes:

> *Many widespread and familiar maladies can masquerade as mental disorders: thyroid disorders, diabetes, Alzheimer's disease and other dementias, sleep apnea and other sleep disorders, temporal lobe epilepsy, HIV, the long-term consequences of head trauma, Lyme disease, and the side effects of medications, to name only a few. These and other physical conditions are common in patients who are seen by mental health practitioners; these medical conditions are also often the very source of the presenting clinical picture.*

Dr. Robert Bransfield is a psychiatrist and noted expert on how Lyme disease affects the brain. He says Lyme-related psychiatric symptoms may start with brain fog and fatigue, progress to anxiety and depression, and eventually lead to major psychiatric disorders such as psychosis and suicide. He characterizes Lyme disease as a brain trauma and notes that it can cause different impairments in different people.

Most research into Lyme and the brain looks at adults, not children. However, in 2001, a study published in the *Journal of Neuropsychiatry and Clinical Neurosciences* compared children with neurological Lyme disease to healthy control subjects. The researchers found that children with Lyme had significantly more cognitive and psychiatric issues. They concluded, "Lyme disease in children may be accompanied by long-term neuropsychiatric disturbances, resulting in psychosocial and academic impairments."

Some children with Lyme exhibit significant anxiety. Some have Attention Deficit Hyperactivity Disorder (ADHD) symptoms that were never present before the child contracted Lyme. Others have symptoms of obsessive-compulsive disorder, lack of impulse control, paranoia and even psychotic symptoms. Many have problems with executive functioning—the set of cognitive processes that allow us to organize, plan, and carry out tasks. Children with Lyme may be highly sensitive to light and sound, or have other sensory issues.

Many have sleep problems. Sleep disturbance, common to Lyme patients, exacerbates many issues—pain, psychiatric symptoms, decline in cognitive and executive functioning, and the inability to stay alert during the day. Furthermore, according to Dr. Bransfield, "Impaired sleep correlates with impaired immune functioning." Parents of children with Lyme need to recognize that sleep problems are not the result of bad sleep habits, but part of the illness itself.

Where does this leave the child with Lyme who needs help dealing with pre-diagnosis Lyme trauma—the result of being dismissed, perhaps verbally abused, and told repeatedly for months or years that there was nothing medically wrong? Where does it leave the mother who is told she is neglectful for letting her child stay home from school when a child can't even get out of bed? Where does this leave a family that is overwhelmed by the illness of the child? Many of these children, adolescents, and parents may desperately need psychotherapy or family counseling.

Mental health practitioners use the *Diagnostic and Statistical Manual of Mental Disorders* for diagnosis, often referred to as the DSM. Published by the American Psychiatric Association, it lists diagnostic criteria for all psychiatric disorders recognized by the United States health care system. The DSM addresses symptoms and syndromes of dysfunction. It does not address the causes of these conditions. In 2015, mental health professionals transitioned from the fourth edition (DSM-IV) to the fifth edition (DSM-5).

At the very least, this DSM diagnosis is needed for the client to receive reimbursement from his medical insurance plan, so it is an important issue. Yet, the DSM presupposes that a set of symptoms adds up to a mental illness diagnosis. In my view, that supposition does not hold true for those who have a medical illness that presents as that set of symptoms. I therefore don't find it appropriate to use a mental illness diagnosis when a medical diagnosis explains the reason for the symptoms. For instance, anxiety, depression, and other symptoms can be caused by Lyme disease, as well as other medical illnesses. Patients who have these symptoms are not mentally ill, but have a medical illness that causes the anxiety or depression.

In the *DSM-5 Made Easy*, by James Morrison, the medical practitioner can find diagnoses that fit the patient who has neuropsychiatric symptoms of tick-borne diseases. For example, if the child with Lyme has anxiety or depression, the appropriate diagnoses might be one of the following:

- F06.4 Anxiety Disorder Due to Another Medical Condition
- F06.31 Depressive Disorder Due to Another Medical Condition with Depressive Features.

These are only two examples of DSM-5 codes that can be used by practitioners to properly indicate that the patient does not have a discrete mental illness, but has psychiatric symptoms from tick-borne diseases. (Note: In the DSM-IV, an appropriate diagnosis for Lyme patients is 293.9—Mental Disorder from a General Medical Condition.)

I recommend that parents ask the practitioner what the diagnosis is and what it means. This will help them understand how the practitioner is viewing the child, and whether Lyme is being considered. If the parent is not comfortable doing that, they might check it out online on a website such as Behavenet.com, which has information about DSM diagnostic codes.

Through years of working with families of children with Lyme disease, I have developed a protocol geared to their complex needs. I tend to work mostly with mothers because typically they are the ones who call and ask me for help. Usually, they are the primary caregivers for their chronically ill children, whether the parents are together or not. I encourage fathers to participate to whatever extent they can. Often they are working long hours to provide for the family while the mother stays home with the child. In some cases, the father is the primary caregiver. And with gay couples, one may be the stay-at-home parent while the other is the primary breadwinner. If the child is able to leave the house, I often work directly with him or her as well.

My approach includes the following:

- Validating the individual experiences of parents and child in their search for a medical diagnosis and treatment. Helping them develop strategies for moving forward.

- Working to build a therapeutic team and foster communication among team members.

- Helping my client—usually the mother of a child with Lyme—deepen her understanding of emotional boundaries. Helping her learn how to use them to maintain healthy and productive relationships, both within and outside of the family. (See Chapter Five on "boundaries")

- Empowering parents to advocate for their family with schools and medical practitioners.

- Helping the chronically ill child foster a personal identity that goes beyond that of a Lyme patient, so that the illness does not define him.

By the time families come to me, they often feel emotionally battered by their experience. They may have lost all confidence in their own ability to handle the situation leaving them feeling hopeless.

Hope Comes First

My first job is to give these parents hope so that they can give their child hope. I help them find a new way to look at the illness and their situation—with schools, doctors, and extended family members. I help them recognize that they don't have to stay stuck in their circumstances. This process begins at our intake session.

Many parents come in focused on the traumatic experiences they have had in their search for someone who could accurately diagnose and treat their child. I suggest that they change the way they think about it. I ask them to consider "Day One" to be when they were diagnosed with Lyme, rather than the day the symptoms began. This new Day One changes everything. We put the trauma on a back burner, and we focus on what it will take to get well. I did that myself in 1990, when I began Lyme treatment. I didn't forget the dark years of searching for answers. However, deciding that my healing journey started on July 9, 1990, the day I was diagnosed, made my burden lighter.

When I meet with a child, my first goal is to give him hope, as well. I help him focus on what he *has* instead of grieving for what he has lost. We discuss what he loves to do, what is still in his life, his dreams and aspirations that are not related to Lyme. Doing otherwise would keep him mired in his debilitating illness, unable to look for the light at the end of the tunnel. Restoring hope, for the parents and child, is the first step in breaking the logjam.

Respect and Choice—With Children and Adults

Respect is another guiding principle of my work. If the child is able to come to my office, I usually meet her in the second session along with her parents. I find that even adolescents feel safer initially in the presence of a parent, usually the mother. Typically, the mother is the child's safety zone. In one case, a girl prefers having both her mother and grandmother in some of her sessions, since her grandmother is a major part of her day-to-day life. Because I want the child to feel comfortable, I include grandma at the child's request.

At my initial meeting with the child, I begin by asking her whether she is comfortable in my office environment. I can give her choices of lighting (natural lighting or one of several lamps. I never use the overhead fluorescents, which can be especially bothersome to people with Lyme disease. Does she prefer the window open or closed? Am I speaking too loudly? What about the temperature of the room— too hot, too cold? Many children with Lyme have sensory issues. I give her choices that can help make the room more comfortable for her.

I then ask why she thinks her parents have brought her to me, and we discuss why I am now in her life. How could the child trust me if I just assumed she understood my role? Would it be respectful of her not to begin with this discussion? Usually, my young clients just listen in the beginning. But some children have a lot to say, and ask a lot of questions. I do my best to answer them. If there is a specific reason why they're coming to see me at this point in time—such as difficulties in school—we discuss that. I say that I will join with her, her parents, and her doctor to form a team to work with the school on figuring out how to help her to learn better.

Sometimes a young child will ask me if I'm a doctor, if I take blood, or give shots. They may assume that if it's about Lyme, I must at least draw blood. Sometimes they don't say a thing when they first come in. So I let them know that I know a lot about Lyme disease, and that what I do is help families who have Lyme figure things out. But I'm not a doctor. I don't draw blood or give shots. I don't even know *how* to do any of that.

Although I have important areas to cover, I know that timing is critical and restraint is vital. I prioritize what the child and family believe to be important and don't throw my ideas in all at once. I want to help them find clarity, not overwhelm them even more. Sometimes, the child or family is at imminent risk. If the child is suicidal, for instance, or exhibiting high-risk behaviors, I'll address that quickly. But for the most part, I wait. Respect and choice are intertwined. Each family has a unique rhythm. Giving parents and children choices—who should be in the session, what we should work on, how often they will see me—shows respect for them and for those rhythms.

Problem Solving is the Cornerstone of the Work

I focus on helping families define and solve problems. Acknowledging that most families have already been through traumatic months or years, when the suffering of the child and family were not taken seriously, is an important start. A key part of my work is helping patients and their families go from being victims, to survivors, to thrivers. If a mother sees herself as a victim, for instance, it's difficult for her to seek solutions. Empowering her to advocate for her child can help bring her out of victimhood.

My intake process actually begins when the parent (usually the mother) calls me. I spend some time on the phone learning about the child's struggles, whether other family members have Lyme as well, and what led the parent to contact me. In the beginning, she may not realize the scope of the help I have to offer. During that first call, I explain what I do—problem solving, defining and protecting boundaries, building the right team of practitioners, helping her navigate a perhaps-contentious relationship with her child's school. When people call, they often don't realize that help in these areas is even possible. After this conversation, if the parent feels that I might be able to help them, she makes an appointment. This process is the beginning of problem solving. The parent schedules an appointment based on solid information about how I can help, rather than going into it blind.

In our sessions, we may talk about how a child or parent felt at various steps along the way, especially how they felt when they finally got the diagnosis. But feelings are not the primary focus of my work, which is to identify problems and move towards solutions. Each family's issues are unique. Some need guidance in how to choose a Lyme-knowledgeable medical practitioner. Many need help dealing with school. Most need help setting boundaries regarding other people in their lives.

Mothers and fathers may have different points of view about medical treatment. When the parents are divorced, there may be a greater disconnect between them. If one doesn't want to talk to me, I may focus on helping the other parent explore solutions to this disagreement. Ideally, the parents will find a way to work together for the benefit of their child.

Empowerment

A thread that runs throughout my work, both with parents and with children, is the concept of empowerment. Empowerment begins with knowledge. I give every new client who comes to my office a "Lyme folder." Inside are articles relevant to their child's particular situation, along with copies of the covers of books that I think will be helpful. I also include one or two issues of *The Lyme Times*, published by LymeDisease.org. I encourage families to join this organization, so they can continue to receive this important source of information about tick-borne diseases, the politics of Lyme, and personal stories that they may be able to relate to.

Next, I help clients clarify where they feel trapped by circumstances and help them figure out how to get free. For instance, attending school for a full day may be a major problem for children with Lyme disease. We examine the family's options, including strategies for dealing with school administrators who may have had little experience with Lyme disease. Each situation is unique, and the work I do is very individualized. It begins with the parent and her prior experience with self-advocacy. Some people find it almost impossible to be assertive with school officials. Helping a mother or father find the strength, knowledge, and courage to stand up for the child's educational needs can be a complicated process.

Often parents have had wonderful experiences dealing with school before their child became ill. They may have volunteered in the classroom, joined the PTA, and communicated well with teachers. Now that the child is ill, the parents expect that cooperation to continue. But all too often, it doesn't. As the child loses ground academically due to Lyme disease, the parents may find themselves in an adversarial position with school authorities. Efforts to help officials understand what's going on may fall on deaf ears. Parents must now learn about their child's educational rights and assert themselves in the school arena. Their child may need vigorous advocacy in order to get the appropriate school supports. I work with mothers and fathers to develop an understanding that being assertive is not the same as being aggressive. And it is so necessary for their child's educational success.

Children need empowerment too. Sometimes it has to do with peers, who may tease them or challenge the very idea of their illness. My young client might say, "Johnny's been my best friend since kindergarten, but he says I can't be that sick because I look good. He doesn't understand why I can't go to school." I'd ask the child: "What does your friend know about Lyme disease? Look at you, you even know what a spirochete is and what probiotics are for!" (I've had little kids describe to me—even better than some adults do—what a spirochete is and even what a herx is and how it affects them.) "You can tell your friend: I'd love to play Legos with you. Can you come over, and we can play? But I don't want to talk about Lyme, my Mom's handling that." Setting that limit can be empowering even to someone who is quite young. The child learns to establish a boundary, something that will come in handy years later in any number of ways.

Children also need empowerment when it comes to talking to adults—grandparents, teachers, parents of friends. I help them with that process by empowering them in the session *with me.* In some cases, we talk about their interests first. One young client plays "Minecraft" and loves to teach me about the game. Another has an outstanding collection of miniature dinosaurs and is knowledgeable about each one. An adolescent taught me about the rise and fall of the Roman Empire, something he learned by watching the History

Channel when he was unable to attend school. We get to issues that are important, directly related to their struggles with Lyme, but it does not have to take up the whole session. The opportunity to teach me about subjects they know well and have a passion for is empowering. It also demonstrates that Lyme is not who they are, but only an illness they are dealing with.

Next I work on empowering the child with her parents. We discuss areas in which she can have a choice (perhaps clothing she wears and, to some extent, food she eats). I help her find her voice in discussing those areas with her parents. Once she can advocate for herself with me and with her parents, it's much easier for her to do so with other adults, as well as with her peers.

Here's an example of a parent and an 8-year-old girl who were at loggerheads over taking medication. The mother would give her daughter the medicine, and the girl would refuse to take it. The mother would insist and the child would dig in her heels even more. It turned into a contest of wills and a screaming match, with neither side listening to the other. When the mother came to me, she was frustrated and worried that, without the medication, her child would not get well. They'd finally found the right doctor, yet she couldn't get her child to cooperate.

I certainly understood the mother's point of view, and then I tried to understand the child's. When I asked why she wouldn't take the medicine, the girl said it tasted awful. She was not simply being oppositional, as it first appeared, but had a genuine aversion to the taste of the medication. I suggested that the mom ask the doctor if there were other options. Might a better tasting alternative antibiotic be appropriate? Or could this medication be ordered through a compounding pharmacy, where it could be flavored differently? The doctor didn't want to change the medication, but had no problem using a compounding pharmacy. In this case, changing the flavor fixed the problem, and the girl now took her medicine without complaint. The daily fights were over. The core problem for the child had been the taste of the medication. What had developed from that was a power struggle that hijacked the parent/child relationship and left them both feeling trapped and helpless. By learning to identify the problem and speak up about it, the girl got her needs met. Both the mother and the child learned the benefits of problem-solving instead of stubbornly refusing to budge.

The Disease Does Not Define the Person

Another aspect of my work with clients is to minimize Lyme in the mindset of the child and family. Coping with the illness takes a large part of every day, with lots of things to think about and lots of problems to solve. But, it does not have to define the individual.

In my first session with a child or adolescent, I focus on connecting with my young client. As I learn about her life, her illness becomes "smaller" in my head. There's more to this young person than Lyme. To help her see that too, and to get away from the constant, overwhelming focus on Lyme disease, I ask about what she enjoys doing. Learning about what the child is like, and what her family is like, helps me consider the whole picture, even as we're dealing with the disease itself.

I ask about the children's pets and tell them about my two cats. (This discussion is particularly interesting for very young patients). They tell me stories about their pets. I don't encourage families to get pets, particularly dogs, since they have to spend time out of doors where they can pick up ticks. However, if pets are already a part of the household, they can be an emotionally safe and therapeutic part of the child's life. Pets don't make a child take his medicine, or go to doctors, or do homework. I discuss that and tell them that it's nice to have "Spot" in the house to turn to, when he's overwhelmed. However, I discuss possible tick exposure from pets that go outside. We talk about strategies for keeping the family, including Spot, safe. I engage the child, even a young one, in trying to solve the problem. I encourage him to talk to his parents, as well as their vet, about options. Being a part of the conversation that seeks solutions can be empowering for a child.

As we get acquainted, I might also learn some other factors that may be directly related to Lyme disease. Does the family live in a wooded area? Do they like to visit nature preserves? As I listen and learn, I am not too quick to suggest major lifestyle changes. For instance, if I told them to get rid of the dog and never go camping or hiking, that could pull the emotional rug out from under them. That would take away pastimes they enjoy. I need to respect the underlying values of their lifestyle choices—family time spent together camping, enjoying and appreciating nature, and learning to care for a pet.

Before I make any such suggestions, I need to explore with them new directions. Day hikes or biking on well-manicured trails. Zoos, aquariums and science museums. A pet that doesn't go outside. They could also develop new hobbies that they can do alone or with others, such as baking, indoor crafts, woodworking, playing or listening to music. Perhaps Minecraft, a video game that is conceptually like Legos, but suitable for kids who have problems with fine motor coordination. Spurred by their need for a special diet, several of my young clients have taken up cooking. They derive great pleasure from seeking out special recipes and preparing family meals.

I know from my own experience that giving up something you love can leave a void. Before contracting Lyme, I was an avid tent camper for 24 years. As my children grew up, we camped in the

Adirondack and Catskill mountains, and along the Finger Lakes and the St. Lawrence Seaway. We visited Yellowstone, Glacier, and other national parks. We lived a half-mile from the Appalachian Trail and would hike parts of it. The day I was diagnosed with Lyme disease, I told my husband that I'd never camp again, and I haven't.

I mourned for the natural beauty of the outdoors, seen close up, from a campsite and a hiking trail, carrying our kayak through the wooded terrain down to a mountain lake. So, I understand and respect how hard it is for patients to forego things that have always given them great joy. It's a process that takes time—and for children and adolescents, it can be much harder than for adults. I work with the child and her parents on recognizing their options, and what the consequences are of maintaining or giving up some of those lifestyle choices. We examine whether stopping something they enjoy might be permanent or temporary and focus on ways to move on.

seven

Responsive Psychotherapy And Lyme Disease

THE LAST CHAPTER GAVE AN OVERVIEW of psychotherapy as it relates to those who have Lyme disease. I help families make sense of their experience and find solutions to their problems. The model I have developed, which I call *responsive psychotherapy*, is non-hierarchical. I don't tell my clients what to do, nor do I sit back and merely reflect their feelings. Together, my clients and I look at their lives and figure out ways to move forward. This is based on how they define their own needs, not on what I determine those needs to be. My goal is to accomplish the following:

- empowerment of the Lyme patient and parents;
- improved communication between parents and within the family as a whole;
- improved advocacy skills in all arenas (medical, educational, and others);
- ability of the parent to understand and enforce boundaries with extended family members and others;

- ability of the parent to set aside emotions in order to do some complex problem-solving, on behalf of the child and family.

I hope this chapter will help parents understand this process, and what these Lyme-affected families should seek from a therapist.

Comprehensive Intake

My initial appointment with the parent takes two hours. I ask for detailed family information about drug and alcohol abuse, as well as mental illness. This is important for several reasons. Is there a pre-existing family tendency toward anxiety, for example? That might help explain why one of the child's presenting Lyme symptoms is anxiety. Knowing this helps us address related problems. Does a family member currently abuse drugs or alcohol, or have an untreated mental illness? Such factors could disrupt the life of the child and family. As we begin to look at Lyme-related issues. Boundaries would need to be set up around the person who, for whatever reason, is not currently stable.

Family Safety

I ask questions to assess the safety of family members. There may be physical violence in the home—a parent who uses corporal punishment on his child, or an older sibling who is abusive. If I see the need, I raise this during the intake.

In the wake of the tragic murder of 20 children at Sandy Hook Elementary School, in Newtown, CT, the town next to mine, I am more vigilant about discussing guns. Does the family own firearms? If so, where are they kept? Are they locked up? Who has the keys? Do the children know where those keys are? I tell them about the impulsivity and mood swings that can accompany Lyme and co-infections. We talk about ways to keep the home safer for the child.

The cabinet should always be locked, with the key kept where the child can't find it. If the child has rages (not unheard of in children with tick-borne diseases), I recommend removing all guns from the home. If a parent belongs to a hunting club, perhaps the weapons can be stored there. Another option may be to keep the guns at the home of a family member or close friend, well-secured. *The child should not know where the guns are.*

It is important to assess any risky behaviors the child with Lyme may exhibit. Does she threaten to harm herself or someone else? Does she talk about dying? If the child seems at high risk of harming herself or anyone else, the parent and I discuss a safety plan. Removing knives and scissors, perhaps. Never leaving the child alone. It may be time for a psychiatrist to evaluate the child for medications. For some children, tick-borne diseases cause a high level of impulsivity. They must be watched closely, so high-risk behaviors can be addressed quickly. Some things cannot wait.

In rare cases, children who are an imminent danger to themselves or others may require psychiatric hospitalization, despite the fact that these symptoms come from the tick-borne disease and not a mental illness. This is truly a last resort, since it will likely interfere with appropriate Lyme treatment. It is almost impossible to find an inpatient psychiatric facility that will allow the child to remain on the antimicrobial medications prescribed by the Lyme doctor.

In the vast majority of cases, the hospital defines the child as mentally ill. No one acknowledges the tick-borne diseases underlying the mood and behaviors. Without an understanding of tick-borne diseases, practitioners may not realize that the symptoms often fluctuate from day to day. They may see the variability as caused by willful behavior. For example, a rage may be triggered by Lyme and co-infections, and not by a child's intention to misbehave. Responding to the child as if the rage was under the child's control can certainly undermine the relationship between the practitioner and the child. This leaves her in an inpatient facility where she feels completely isolated.

For many patients, Lyme is an invisible disability. Because these children do not look sick, many people, including medical professionals, may doubt that they are physically ill.

They may be taken off of the Lyme medications and put on psychotropic medications that don't address the true source of their symptoms. Furthermore, based on the mistaken diagnosis, an insurance company may deny further treatment for Lyme disease. I strive to keep children with Lyme disease out of psychiatric facilities, if at all possible, unless it is unsafe to do so.

What About Lyme Disease?

Once we've completed the family history, we can finally begin to look at Lyme. My focus differs from that of a medical doctor. I'm not concerned with blood work or most other diagnostic reports. I look at how the child and family are coping with the illness, how they make decisions, and how Lyme impacts the way they function.

As we talk about Lyme, I ask about the child's symptoms and when they started. A picture emerges of the family's Lyme journey, from the beginning of symptoms, through the months or years of searching for a doctor to determine what is wrong, to the diagnosis, beginning of treatment, and up to the point of this intake session with me. Every family's experience is different. However, in more than 20 years of seeing children with Lyme disease, I find one overwhelming commonality. Most families that I have seen vividly recall feeling abused by practitioners who told them that there was nothing wrong with their child. They may have also been told that the child or mother was mentally ill. Many children and parents feel wounded by this experience, and I can help them get past that. My work helps to prevent post-traumatic stress disorder (PTSD) symptoms. We deal with the trauma earlier rather than much later, when symptoms suggestive of PTSD may solidify. But that's generally not the work I need to do immediately.

During the intake, I ask the parent to look with me to an earlier time. What was her child like before Lyme symptoms began, sometimes years before diagnosis? What was his temperament? Was he calm and easy, or edgy and aggressive? Often, parents tell me that the mood swings, behavior problems, and rages began at a discrete point in time, sometimes with the onset of physical symptoms.

If the child is not doing well in school, I want to know when those problems started, as well. Was he an attentive student with no complaints from teachers until his grades or behavior took a nosedive? If so, the school-related issues may have actually been the first symptoms, well before the onset of physical manifestations like headaches or joint pain.

Parents of children who have had Lyme symptoms from early childhood may not even know what *normal* is. Let's say a child is diagnosed at age 13. However, as a toddler she didn't sleep well, was sensitive to light and sound at age 5, and had trouble learning to read once she was in school. All of these seemingly disparate symptoms may have been signs of Lyme disease. Thus, there may be no *normal* for the child or parents to refer back to.

This information about background in mood, behaviors, and school performance sets the stage for the work we need to do. I ask about other family members. Does anyone else have Lyme? Does anyone have symptoms that might be undiagnosed Lyme? Is there a sibling with "learning issues?" At this point, I don't generally delve into the possibility of Lyme in undiagnosed siblings. I don't want to overwhelm the parent. However, I do note the learning issues as a possible indicator that the diagnosed child may not be the only family member with Lyme.

In the final part of the intake, we look at issues requiring our immediate attention. Although every family is different, school is usually a big concern. Complaints typically include failing grades, spotty attendance, or behavior problems. Some parents are very worried about the social isolation that comes with the illness. Perhaps their child is unwilling or unable to keep in touch with friends. Other parents may be apprehensive about intrusive relatives who are planning to visit soon.

What About the Pre-Diagnosis Trauma?

The process of getting to a Lyme diagnosis can be very traumatic. Lyme patients and their families may be misunderstood, dismissed, insulted, and belittled. They may be accused of lying, malingering, or suffering from a mental illness. Parents may be charged with abuse or neglect. This pre-diagnosis trauma is often one of the most important issues to be addressed in psychotherapy. Consider the following case.

Fifteen-year-old Joanie had been ill for some time. Severe pain kept her awake at night. It prevented her from taking part in daily activities, such as school, sports, and sometimes even eating dinner with her family. Often, she was confined to bed. When the search for a diagnosis had been fruitless, her primary care doctor had recommended an inpatient pain management program. Unbeknownst to her parents, the doctors and therapists in this program considered Joanie's pain to be psychosomatic.

The inpatient program did nothing to diminish her pain since, as the family would eventually learn, it was caused by undiagnosed Lyme disease. Now home from the hospital and receiving Lyme treatment, Joanie was experiencing dangerous episodes of rage that threatened her safety and that of her family. She directed most of this fury at her mother. While I counseled the mother, Joanie saw an outpatient therapist who knew nothing about Lyme but was willing to learn. I was brought in to provide clinical consultation on the case.

In my view, at least some of Joanie's out-of-control behavior came from the trauma of her inappropriate hospital treatment. I helped Joanie's therapist recognize how deeply such misdiagnosis and mistreatment can affect Lyme patients. Yet, Lyme encephalopathy (disorder or disease of the brain) can cause behavioral problems, including rages. So, it wasn't clear how much of the out-of-control behavior was due to Lyme, and how much was due to the trauma of the past year.

As I saw it, we needed to help Joanie understand the level of betrayal and abuse she had experienced. Working with her therapist, I learned that this teenager had suppressed her feelings while trapped in the hospital. Her anger toward the professionals in the hospital had built up. I speculated that she had displaced it onto her parents. Furthermore, Joanie felt betrayed by her parents because they had taken her to the hospital in the first place. Together Joanie and her therapist looked at the betrayal and abuse, and clarified what had really happened. They jointly acknowledged how each professional at the hospital had contributed to the reign of terror that had surrounded this girl during her lengthy hospital stay.

With the help of her therapist, Joanie started to see her experience in a different light. As she became appropriately angry at the hospital, her fury towards her parents diminished. As she addressed these issues in therapy, Joanie's behavior at home improved. She was no longer at risk of harming someone else or herself. There was still Lyme encephalopathy. But the rage that stemmed from the trauma of the hospitalization appeared to have dissipated. As Joanie freed herself from the damage that experience had inflicted on her, she felt much safer in her home and in the world around her. As I had suspected, in this case, the trauma needed direct and immediate psychotherapeutic intervention.

Keeping Multiple Tracks in My Head at the Same Time

This principle bears some explaining. It is vital to the success of therapy with a chronic Lyme patient. As I follow one track with a client—one line of inquiry, one train of thought—I consider other paths we may want or need to pursue at a later time. For instance, perhaps I am seeing a parent about a serious school-related issue. As we roll up our sleeves to address that problem, I am mindful of other concerns. Should we document the child's impairments with a neuropsychological evaluation? How should we address his sleep problems? Might he have vision problems, which would require a full examination by a neuro-optometrist? As important as these questions are, I must weigh whether it would be useful to bring them up now or wait a while. I don't want to overwhelm the parent, who already feels burdened. Another track I often keep in mind is whether other family members might have undiagnosed Lyme. Unless there has been a recent tick bite, however, I typically don't bring up that question right away.

The Life of the Family With Lyme

A family with Lyme has unique dynamics. The ailing child may be angry, particularly with his mother. After all, shouldn't parents protect their children? The child may feel betrayed because his mother did not quickly solve the problem when he first became ill. Instead, she took him from doctor to doctor, who may have accused him of lying or malingering. He may have been misdiagnosed and given medications that didn't work or caused more suffering.

Other family members may be angry, as well. The stress of caring for their seriously ill child and the frustrating search for answers may be contributing to long-simmering antagonism between the parents. Siblings may resent all the attention the sick child receives and may feel neglected. This anger needs to be recognized, validated when appropriate and dealt with. In my experience, having the child and family talk about it can help. When they come to realize that they have all been betrayed by a system that fails to understand Lyme, the anger among family members dissipates. Together with the child and family, we leave the anger behind and return to problem-solving mode—right where we need to be.

Many children with Lyme tell me how isolated and hopeless they feel. They are confused and scared. Then there is the way that doctors view the mothers (less so, the fathers). When the treatment plan for the wrong diagnosis doesn't work, doctors may look with suspicion at the mother, in most families the child's primary caregiver. Doctors may presume that the mother isn't following the treatment plan, which may include ordering the child to return to school immediately. A doctor may refuse to write a note to school stating that the child requires homebound instruction, even if the child is too sick to get out of bed.

Doctors may presume that the child has school phobia, separation anxiety, or some other blaming type of a diagnosis. In rare cases, doctors may even report mothers for neglect because the student is not in school. Or they may assert that the mother has "Munchausen's by Proxy," assuming that the mother is making the child ill to get attention for herself. In case of divorce, the parent who agrees with the medical establishment may deny that the child's symptoms are due to a physical illness. The Lyme-denying parent may even be granted full custody of the child, with only supervised visitation for the other parent. Investigations by child protective agencies can even lead to removal of the child to foster care.

Putting it All Together—How I Work

I saw Julia for the intake. She was eager for me to see her 10-year-old daughter, Cynthia, who had regressed both physically and emotionally a few months after a tick bite. Cynthia now sucked her thumb, which she hadn't done in years. She had daily headaches, night terrors, and started wetting the bed. According to her mother, Cynthia also seemed to have lost her confidence. "She doesn't want to see her friends. She used to be such an outgoing, happy child." After many doctors failed to identify the problem, a Lyme specialist diagnosed her with tick-borne diseases and began treatment.

Since the mother also had Lyme, I explained that I wanted to help her identify her own goals. She needed to get her own confidence back and begin to solve some of the problems that had emerged since her family had become ill. Julia and I had a few sessions before she and I felt it was time for me to meet Cynthia.

Cynthia came in with her Mom. In most cases, a child with Lyme needs the comfort of her mother's presence when she comes for counseling. Unless the child requests to see me alone, I never see a young child without her parent. I honor the attachment between a child who is ill and her mother—the source of security, comfort, and emotional healing.

Often when a mother comes to see me, she brings up the issue of the close tie she has to her child. Others, including doctors and mental health professionals, have told her that she's *too close* to her child. The child is, after all, no longer a baby or toddler. They tell the mother to let go, to get out more, to work on her own life. They accuse her of being overprotective, even "enmeshed" with her child, of interfering with her child's emotional growth. The mother cannot bring herself to move away from her child. But she feels intensely guilty, since the professionals are telling her to let go.

I don't agree. In my view, Julia needs to stay right where she is. That attachment that is so healthy and vital for growth between the mother and the newborn baby, that symbiosis, can also be the foundation for wellbeing and growth in an older child who is traumatized. When a child becomes gravely ill, returning to that early bond with the mother provides emotional safety. Within the warmth of that bond, the child is more likely to comply with medical treatment, take her medications, and go to school if she is able. This is because she feels that her mother is with her every step of the way. Without that, the child is left alone, isolated, and in many cases, even more terrified than she is by the illness itself.

I ask Cynthia what Mom has told her about why she is meeting with me. Cynthia shrugs her shoulders and doesn't say much. So, I go on. Making her feel comfortable in my office and in my presence is my job, not hers. Pressuring either a child or parent to speak is not how I work. I am not there to add to anyone's burden.

Cynthia is quite ill. I bring up Lyme disease right away, rather than asking her about what she likes to do, as I would with more talkative children. Those who are very quiet when they come in often cannot tolerate a full hour's session. So I get to the point, not knowing when her fatigue may shut her down completely. It's important to keep in mind that the fatigue of Lyme has been shown in controlled studies to be the equivalent of the fatigue in congestive heart failure, so I take it very seriously.

"Cynthia," I say, "I know a lot about Lyme disease, especially how it affects kids. Mom has brought you here to talk to me about Lyme and what it's like for you. My job is to help you while you're living with Lyme, with whatever problems you and your Mom want to talk about—in your family, in school, or wherever."

I go on. "I'd like you to know that I had Lyme disease. It made me feel sick every day. I finally found the right doctor, took medicine for a long time, and got well. When I figured out what was wrong with me and started to get well, I decided to help other people while they were going through the same thing."

Cynthia perks up, even begins to smile. At that moment, my connection with her has begun—10 or 15 minutes into that session. It's not only the fact that I had Lyme that forms the connection, it's how I tell her about it. I choose my words carefully. Hearing about my own experience with Lyme helps Cynthia realize that I understand what she's going through. As always, my goal is to show her that someone understands, and offer hope that she will get well.

Then, I ask her about her headaches, stomach aches and how she is sleeping—concrete symptoms she can easily identify. She tells me about her daily headaches. I talk to her about how bad they are. When children are in pain, they *always* experience the pain as bad. So I don't ask if the headaches are sometimes mild, or use a ten-point rating system. I use language appropriate to her age. I ask Cynthia, "Some days, are they terrible, and other days, are they worse than terrible? Are there any days when your head doesn't hurt, or you hardly notice it? She goes on to describe her headaches—what part of the head, how bad they get, time of day.

I'm not her doctor. I don't assess the quality, quantity or origin of the headaches, or develop a medical treatment plan. Rather, I'm the "Lyme lady." I'm the one Cynthia can talk to about what she is living with, day after day. She needs to feel that I am safe to talk to, and believe that I can help her define and solve problems as they come along. She has already been to many practitioners with whom she did not feel emotionally safe. Perhaps thinking she was malingering, these doctors told her parents to ignore the headaches, and make her do her chores and homework anyway. They said Cynthia's headaches were psychosomatic and that she should see a psychiatrist.

In this first session with Cynthia, we now have two points of connection—the fact that I had Lyme and that I understand her daily, debilitating headaches. I ask about her Lyme doctor and support her relationship with him, saying "Guess what? Dr. Parker sees a lot of kids with Lyme and knows a lot about what medicine to use to make those headaches go away!"

Again, I don't speak as the medical expert. A child needs confidence in her doctor and in the choices her Mom and Dad make for her. That confidence and trust help build hope in the child that she can get well. It also supports compliance with treatment.

When I ask Cynthia about school, she gets quiet. I assume that she feels embarrassed because she's not doing well in school. So again, I take the lead. "Some kids with Lyme have a really hard time with school," I say. "Lyme seems to slow down a kid's brain. It's hard to hear everything the teacher says. And it's *really hard* to answer all the questions on a test." Cynthia engages again. She tells me about an exam that was hard to understand and how she hates being called on in class.

I tell her again that Lyme does that to people. "Do you want to hear the good news, Cynthia?" She nods. "Those medications you're taking can get rid of the Lyme in your brain and help you think better. It can take a long time, but then it can happen. You can answer the teacher's questions, at least some of the time. You can finish your test. The clouds in your brain are gone!" She's relieved, and we have another point of connection between us.

I've made some mistakes along the way. Once, I talked to a young child about the "bugs in his brain." He got really upset, imagining bugs crawling around. I never said that again!

My initial goal with a child is to develop points of connection. I let her know that I understand her situation, and I anchor our relationship in facts. I never talk down to a child.

Often school is troubling to both the parent and child. In that case, I talk about how I can help. "Cynthia, there are a lot of kids all over the country who have Lyme disease and have problems with school," I say. "I'm really glad you told me what you're having the most trouble with. Your parents and I can work on figuring out how to make it better." That's all the child needs to know in the first session.

Cynthia and I are connected. We've started the work. I don't define her as having a "job" in seeking solutions to the problems. But, I reinforce her role by asking her to tell me what goes on. By identifying her specific problems, she helps me, as well as her parents to figure out her educational needs and how best to meet them.

I'd like to discuss two specific cases that illustrate how I work with families facing serious challenges.

Case #1—Child Protective Services Investigation

Several years ago, I received a frantic call from the mother of an 11-year-old girl with Lyme disease. After a disagreement with the school district over her child's medical diagnosis, the family was being investigated by Child Protective Services. She feared her daughter would be removed from their home and put into foster care. Because of the urgent situation, I asked to see both the mother and the father for an intake appointment. I was relieved to find that they were absolutely on the same page.

It was a troubling scenario. Because of the girl's profound fatigue and daily fevers, her Lyme doctor said she was too ill to go to school. However, the school did not accept the doctor's opinion. Although this girl had daily fevers of over 101 degrees, her parents were told to send her to school anyway. (I was astonished! Shouldn't parents keep their children home from school when they have a fever?) Yet, school personnel did not believe the family or their Lyme doctor. They wanted the girl evaluated by a school-appointed psychiatrist. Since the parents knew of several families of children with Lyme who took their children to the school's recommended psychiatrist, they agreed. They didn't realize that this fateful decision would haunt them for a long time to come.

To the family's dismay, the psychiatrist wrote in his report that Lyme disease was not the cause of this girl's problems. Instead, he diagnosed her with anxiety and a litany of phobias. The psychiatrist ordered a long list of treatments that were in direct conflict with what the child's Lyme physician had prescribed. Acting in what they believed to be the best interest of their daughter, the parents continued to follow their own doctor's directions. They didn't want to change a treatment plan that was working for their child. And they did not want to follow the advice of a psychiatrist who denied her medical illness.

At that point, school officials filed a complaint with Child Protective Services (CPS). Upon investigation, CPS began taking steps toward removing the child from the home. Child protective workers are not trained to understand the medical complexities of Lyme disease. They may also not be aware that schools, in most cases, are supposed to follow the orders of the child's licensed physician concerning medical issues. Therefore, it's not appropriate for them to make such drastic decisions in such a case. Unfortunately, parents of children with Lyme disease have had similar run-ins with CPS agencies, in various parts of the country.

I was appalled by this entire process. Why would a psychiatrist develop a treatment plan for a child who had been diagnosed with a complex medical illness without even contacting the treating physician? Why would the psychiatrist presume to know when or whether a child with that illness was well enough to attend school? Why wouldn't the psychiatrist consult the child's doctor, who understood the psychiatric manifestations of tick-borne diseases?

When a family is in crisis, my role as a therapist is first, to deal with the crisis. Next, I build a team of Lyme-knowledgeable professionals to gain an understanding of what's going on. Finally, I engage with the parents and the child in problem-solving. In this case, I referred the child to a Lyme-knowledgeable psychiatrist for evaluation. This specialist found that the girl did not have school phobia or an anxiety disorder. He found her symptoms to be consistent with tick-borne diseases, and saw the first psychiatrist's treatment plan was inappropriate. The parents submitted his psychiatric evaluation to CPS.

CPS disregarded the findings of the Lyme expert and accepted those of the school's consulting psychiatrist, who said the child was mentally ill. Because the parents were unwilling to drag their child out of bed to participate in therapies that the first psychiatrist recommended, CPS considered the parents to be "non-compliant." The agency went forward with its plan to remove the child from her home, and the family's nightmare continued.

Then one day, the mother called with good news. CPS had dropped the case because the school's consulting psychiatrist would not testify against the parents. This left the agency without its key—

and perhaps only—witness. We don't know why the doctor refused to go to family court. However, for this family, the legal battle was over.

Case #2—High-risk Behavior

Suzanne and her four children had all suffered from Lyme disease for many years without at first knowing what it was. Once diagnosed, the family's road to recovery had been slow, with many ups and downs. She and I had worked together via the telephone over a period of about three years. When everybody had improved substantially, Suzanne stopped therapy, feeling she could move on without my help.

Then, about a year later, she asked for another phone session. She and her three older children were continuing to do well, but 11-year-old Joey, her youngest, had serious academic problems. It soon became apparent to me that this was due to two important factors. First, although he had an Individualized Education Plan, the school did not appear to understand the type of specialized instruction and accommodations he needed. They repeatedly told Suzanne that he was doing "fine," even as he fell further and further behind. Secondly, I became convinced that he needed a new neuropsychological evaluation, to determine his current deficits in cognition and executive functioning. The previous one had been done four years earlier.

Unlike a learning disability that a child is born with (like dyslexia), Lyme-induced cognitive deficits can wax and wane, just as the headaches and joint pains do. Suzanne and I discussed how to move the school along in meeting Joey's needs. But we also talked about bringing Joey across the country from their home state to New York City. I wanted him to be evaluated by a Lyme-knowledgeable neuropsychologist. Suzanne readily agreed.

135

As we discussed logistics and came closer to putting a plan in place, Suzanne's anxiety began to dissipate. As I said earlier, engaging in problem solving can help a parent come out of victimhood and no longer feeling trapped. In almost all cases, identifying the problem, figuring out what to do about it, and taking steps to put a plan in place will help the parent become more grounded and less anxious.

Then, a crisis erupted. Joey had been hanging out with peers his mother did not approve of, kids who had been in trouble in school and the community. As a result, Suzanne took away Joey's cell phone. Joey had reacted by running away, something he'd never done before. Ever.

I spent a lot of time on the phone with Suzanne and her husband in what was now crisis problem solving. Should the police be contacted? When Lyme is not an issue, I always recommend notifying police when a child has run away. But Lyme complicates things immensely. Police and social services may not recognize the medical illness beneath the behavior. Contacting these agencies that don't know Lyme could be harmful to the child and family, sometimes leading to the involvement of the juvenile justice or legal system. Suzanne knew this from her years of researching Lyme and hearing of problems other parents had faced.

At first, Suzanne and her husband decided not to call the police. Instead, with the help of the older siblings and several family friends, they started searching for Joey. Someone spotted him, but he refused to come home and again ran away from family and friends. This was so out of character for this child! Finally, the parents contacted the police, who located Joey and brought him home.

Before we could determine how to respond to Joey's behavior, we needed to understand more about what was going on with him. What precisely were we dealing with? Was it the kind of oppositional behavior that sometimes arises when a child enters adolescence? He had never acted out like this before. Was it triggered by underlying infection? Joey had been off of antibiotic treatment for Lyme disease and co-infections for over a year at this point. Was this a recurrence of Lyme or bartonella? Or perhaps PANS/PANDAS, a neuropsychiatric condition that brings extreme, sudden changes in behavior? For children with Lyme, behavioral manifestations are often intertwined with other symptoms of the illness.

Luckily, Suzanne and her husband were able to take Joey to the East Coast to see his old Lyme specialist, Dr. Foster.[1] On the same trip, they also scheduled a neuropsychological evaluation with Dr. Kramer,[2] the specialist Suzanne and I had previously discussed. Suzanne kept in touch with me as Joey's journey unfolded, including flights delayed by weather. I worked with her on how to discuss with Joey why he was making the trip, what we hoped to accomplish, and why it mattered so much. Children need to understand what the plans are, and why, particularly when those plans may change quickly. How and what is said to the child is really important. When children understand the plan, even if they don't agree with it, they feel safer. Seeing that their parents are on top of the situation reassures them. Joey was cooperative, though exhausted, by the time they reached New York.

I heard from Suzanne after Joey had seen his Lyme specialist. Dr. Foster confirmed my suspicions that bartonella and perhaps PANS/PANDAS were responsible for Joey's behavior. Following an updated medical history and a thorough physical exam, Dr. Foster made a clinical diagnosis of Lyme and bartonella, ordered blood tests, and prescribed medication. Dr. Foster theorized that a new tick bite had triggered Joey's extreme, sudden change in behavior and

---

1 Not real name
2 Not real name

cognitive decline. Because they caught it early, Dr. Foster believed that there was a good chance Joey would respond well, and treatment would be short.

The second reason for the trip east was for the neuropsychological evaluation. Dr. Kramer found impairments in planning, decision-making, and impulse control consistent with what she had seen in other children with Lyme, bartonella, and even PANS/PANDAS. She also determined that Joey had neuro-optometric problems, and referred him to a specialist for that.

I had speculated that bartonella and possibly PANS/PANDAS were behind Joey's serious behavioral changes. Now, two leading experts, who evaluated him in different ways, had reached the same conclusion. Our team worked on a plan to give Joey the medical treatment he needed, as well as educational supports at school. In addition, a neuro-optometrist prescribed prism glasses, which significantly improved Joey's ability to read. This also made him better at sports, since he could now see what he was doing and react more quickly. This was great news for someone who had been a gifted athlete.

Special Challenges of Divorced and Blended Families

Parents come to see me because of my expertise in working with families who have Lyme disease. They do not seek me out primarily for marriage counseling or to explore how their blended family functions. However, because that is part of their current situation and their history, I look at it during the intake. If things are running smoothly, we just cover the basics. But sometimes problems arise when parents are divorced or when a stepparent and step-siblings enter a family. I look at the rhythm of the family in order to assess whether there is work we need to do. Often there is none. In some cases, even after a contentious divorce, parents are getting along now. Or, one parent willingly takes a back seat when it comes to managing matters of health care and education. However, when the divorced parents are at odds, I will address it. I may invite the parent who doesn't live with the child full-time to come in for some sessions, to learn more about how Lyme disease is affecting the child's life. As needed, I may also involve the stepparent.

Here's one example. Robby, an articulate 10-year-old, was quite ill, although you wouldn't know it to look at him. He lived with his mother, stepfather, and younger half-sister in Connecticut. Robby had a good relationship with his stepfather. Sometimes his stepdad joined in my sessions with Robby and his Mom.

Robby's parents had been divorced for years. His father lived two hours away in New York City, and Robby visited his Dad every few weeks for an overnight, or a weekend. Although told about his son's illness, Robby's father didn't seem interested in details. This became a problem when Mom found out that Robby often skipped his medications when he visited his father. She discussed this with her ex-husband, who said he didn't think it mattered if Robby missed a dose or two. Mom told him that interrupting Robby's treatment protocol could harm their son's chance of recovery, but it didn't seem to make an impression. The situation also troubled Robby. He knew he needed help remembering to take his medications. He also didn't want to be the reason his parents argued.

I suggested that Mom and Robby invite Dad in for a session, and that Robby's stepdad not come to that appointment. They agreed. I suggested that Mom let him know that this was only to learn more about Robby's illness and ways to help their son.

When Dad came in with Robby and his Mom, I focused on concrete problem solving. I did not touch issues related to the divorce or anything that was not connected to Lyme disease and Robby's struggles. It only took one session. Dad understood and began to support Robby's treatment. Things improved between the former spouses, and Robby no longer felt caught in the middle.

Some divorces leave parents angry, arguing, and engaged in power struggles for years. The stress of having a child with Lyme disease adds to the rancor between them. Although their child desperately needs support, they have difficulty coming together to make medical and educational decisions. Sometimes the parents argue over money. After all, treating chronic Lyme disease can be very expensive. Occasionally, these disputes between parents cannot be resolved. However, in many cases, strategies can be developed to bring the parents together to help their child.

Divorced parents who aren't getting along often blame each other, as they may have done during their marriage. This gets in the way of solving problems. Often, but not always, the child lives with the mom. She's in the trenches with medical appointments and school-related issues. So, typically, that's where I begin my work. In these cases, when I see the mom alone first for the intake, I look for ways to help her reduce the level to which she blames the dad. Lessening the intensity of bad feelings between the parents can help bring them together to make important decisions about the child they both love. Recognizing power struggles and working to eliminate the tug of war can help.

I don't try to solve the full scope of the problems between the parents, because that's not why they came to see me. I don't entertain the complaints one has about the other's new spouse or visitation issues, unless it is relevant to the family's challenges with tick-borne diseases. It's easy for a therapist to drift into these other matters, which certainly may be important. But my experience and my Lyme professional education tell me that approach is wrong. The father has agreed to come in to talk about the child's health and school issues. If I move into other arenas, it appears as if I have brought him in under false pretenses. In fact, that would betray one of my guiding principles—respect for boundaries.

I keep it concrete. We discuss the illness, its symptoms and how it impacts the child's ability to function at home and at school. (Hardest for those who haven't researched Lyme to understand are the neuropsychiatric manifestations.) I answer any questions the father might have, to the best of my ability. And I try to bring the parents together to figure out how they can best help their child.

Blended families come with unique histories, family dynamics, and challenges. There may be two sets of parents, with the child's time split between two families. A stepparent may come to the marriage with or without children. One or more children may be the product of the new marriage. It can be quite complicated, even apart from Lyme-related issues.

In my intake, I ask about the particular circumstances of the blended family. How do the parents, stepparents, and children all get along? How involved is each parent in the life of the child who is ill? Are extended family members present in the lives of the family? If so, do they accept the Lyme diagnosis? This helps me see the larger picture.

A couple from New Jersey came to see me. Each had two children, all teenagers, from previous marriages. Shortly after they'd married a few years earlier, Mom's now-13-year-old daughter, Sally, became seriously ill with Lyme disease. She was too sick to attend school. They wanted my help in figuring out how to move forward with medical care, with her education, with her enormous problems with sleep, and other symptoms. Since they had a large family and their marriage was pretty new, I had a number of questions in my mind. How connected was Sally to her stepdad? How strong was this marriage in the face of this crisis? How was it affecting the whole family? Since there didn't seem to be a problem, I left it alone, but kept it in mind as therapy with Sally began.

Mom came with Sally to most sessions. Occasionally a grandparent would bring Sally, if Mom was not available. One time, neither Mom nor Sally's grandparents could come, so her stepdad brought her. When they arrived, I asked Sally whether she wanted to see me alone or invite her stepdad to join us. She told me it was okay to include him. Although I told her that she could at any time ask him to leave if she wanted to talk with me privately, she allowed him to stay for the whole time. Sally's stepdad was very engaged in the session, and it was great having him there. I could see that Sally was comfortable with him, and that the two of them had a good relationship. The fact that a teenager this ill would allow her stepfather into her session said a lot to me. And the respect he demonstrated towards her spoke volumes. I believed their blended family was working out fine.

Complex Support Systems

During my intake, I ask about the family's support system. Are they close to their extended family members? Who in their extended family understands what the child and family are going through? Do their relatives provide support, and if so, what kind? Families that live close by often help out in tangible ways, and some who live at a distance may provide valuable emotional support. (When I was fighting Lyme, my brother and sister-in-law were very helpful, even though they live thousands of miles away. I could talk to them at any time, and they always believed me. When I felt trapped, they often came up with suggestions that helped break the logjam. I never needed to hold back, fearing that what I said would, in some way, be used against me.)

When extended families are not supportive or undermine the parents' decisions, I know I need to delve deeper. Boundary issues need to be examined more closely. What limits should be set with those relatives to protect the child and family? Some relatives can be kept close, while others must be held at arm's length.

Faith-Based Communities

Some families have close faith communities. They consider their congregations to be like family. They've been part of each other's personal lives for years, with everyone feeling welcome and safe. However, when Lyme disease emerges and the child may be unable to attend school, the feeling of closeness and safety within that community may change. So this is an area where I ask more questions.

Sometimes, community members continue to be very supportive. They may offer to cook, clean, or shop, while realizing and acknowledging how overwhelmed the family's life is. They believe the child and parents, and are ready to listen. Unfortunately, that is not always the case. The same tight fellowship that provides the congregation with cohesiveness may isolate the child and family. Some group members may accept incorrect information spread by someone who "doesn't believe in" chronic Lyme. In that case, some parents succeed in educating their congregation. Others may feel compelled to seek out another congregation where they find a new home, a new community. I explore these options with the parents so they can once again feel safe and move forward.

Parenting Strategies—Making a Paradigm Shift

When people become parents, they develop values and practices about the best way to bring up their children. Ideally, these values are agreed upon by both parents and form a structure for family life. Families have their own ways of handling meals, bedtimes, and how much television and video game time is permitted. Families also have their own approach to school. For example, some place more emphasis on academic achievement than others. Many of these routines may be turned upside down when Lyme enters the picture.

Many parents have a hard time realizing that changes in the child's brain can make it difficult for him to follow the usual order of things. Children may develop food aversions, for instance, a result of how Lyme affects the brain. A parent cannot and should not make the child eat a food that he finds disgusting. A power struggle over food doesn't lead to compliance, it just undermines the relationship between the parent and child. And that food aversion may, in fact, be caused by sensory sensitivities common to children with Lyme.

Sleep is another area that can lead to power struggles between parent and child. Psychiatrist Robert Bransfield says Lyme-related sleep problems are not behavioral issues but, rather, a complex aspect of the disease. Some patients have a hard time falling asleep. Others have sleep disturbances during the night (including intrusive thoughts). Some wake up suddenly during the night and remain awake. Sometimes the only way to meet the child's need for restorative sleep is with the use of medication or supplements. In the absence of treatment, many children simply cannot get enough sleep. Arguing over bedtime helps no one. Expecting children with Lyme disease to conform to normal bedtimes is a recipe for frustration.

Battles between parents and children often involve school, primarily attendance, and homework. A child's cognitive impairments and sleep problems may make it impossible to do academic work. Recognize this and work with the school to get an appropriate education plan for a student who is ill. This is far more productive than pushing a child to do what he simply cannot do.

All of these factors leave parents out on a limb. They have structured family life in a certain way for years, and it has worked well. But now with Lyme, many find that what they did before no longer works. They do not know what to do.

I ask them to view parenting decisions in light of their child's illness. If the child had a broken leg, would they expect her to run a footrace? Or even walk across the street? Pushing a child to do what she's incapable of doing damages the relationship between the parent and child. It diminishes the child's perception of the parent as a source of comfort and safety. What serves a child best, in these situations, is for parents to move out of their comfort zone. They may find it hard to base their decisions on the needs of their child, rather than on the patterns they implemented when they started their family. But doing so is vital to their child's recovery.

Co-Morbidity—Lyme and Mental Illness?

I don't discount the possibility that a child with Lyme disease might also be mentally ill. However, in most cases, treating Lyme and co-infections needs to come first. After treatment, the practitioner can focus on whatever psychiatric symptoms may remain. I have developed a way of working that keeps both possibilities in mind. The psychiatric symptoms might be caused by tick-borne diseases, or they may result from unrelated mental illness. I work with the parents to develop strategies to help their child cope, no matter what the root cause.

For example, a child might have severe anxiety. Is it due to Lyme or to a discrete mood disorder? So, I talk to both the parents and the child about the symptoms, reminding them that Lyme treatment might clear up the problem. However, since it's hard to live with severe anxiety, we discuss measures that may help for the time being. One option would be to take the child to a psychiatrist familiar with Lyme to be assessed for medication. Another choice might be a naturopathic doctor, who can suggest dietary supplements that might help. I stress that the child may not need any of the meds or supplements after Lyme symptoms have resolved. We also try to figure out what triggers the anxiety and come up with ways to diminish it. For instance, if the child is afraid of the dark, keep a light on in her bedroom at night—not merely a nightlight, but a lamp. If she can't tolerate the noise and activity on the school bus, drive her to school or arrange a ride, if that is possible. If he becomes anxious after too long a stretch in the classroom, arrange for some decompression time in the school nurse's office. These are survival mechanisms for the short run, as you work towards a long-term resolution of symptoms.

I don't generally recommend behavior modification programs for a child with Lyme disease. In the case of brain dysfunction due to tick-borne illness, the psychiatric symptoms are not behavioral. They are caused by a brain infection, similar to what we see in children with traumatic brain injuries following a car crash. Therapy methods must fit the needs of the patient. The patient shouldn't be expected to fit into the constraints of any specific modality.

Parenting a child with psychiatric symptoms is difficult and complicated. Yet, it's important to recognize that at least some of the child's problems may stem from a treatable medical illness. This can bring hope to parents as they ride this emotional rollercoaster.

eight

Building A Team

Sandy:

WHEN I DISCUSS WITH PARENTS the need to build a team of
practitioners to help their child, I often use the image of a tent on top
of a mountain. The tent alone would not protect us from the winds
and rain. We need to stake it down, dig a trench around it, and keep
it zipped up if the weather is bad. When we take those actions, the
tent that had appeared so fragile is now strong enough to resist bad
weather. We are safe and protected inside our shelter.

When a family comes to me, they may feel as fragile as the
campers in that mountain tent. Building a team is like staking down
the tent. It provides a way to get the support and stability needed to
weather the storms of dealing with Lyme disease.

Tanya sounded overwhelmed. She and her husband and their
son, Josh, all had Lyme disease. Not only was her whole family ill, but
she herself seemed cognitively impaired. She had trouble finding
words for what she wanted to say, as well as problems focusing and

retaining information. Tanya had graduated from college with a degree in science. Since she reported no problems with her college coursework, I didn't think she had a lifelong learning disability. Her current cognitive difficulties and fatigue were typical of many Lyme patients.

Despite her own problems, Tanya's main concern was for her 9-year-old son, Josh. A few months earlier, the family had moved from Minnesota to New York. Then, the whole family had been diagnosed with Lyme disease. Thus, Josh was undergoing the ups and downs of Lyme treatment at the same time he was trying to adjust to the fourth grade at a new school. It was not going well.

Back in Minnesota, Josh had been found to have significant problems with fine motor coordination. Given a special education classification of "other health impaired" (OHI), he had worked with an occupational therapist. Although the OHI designation had followed him to New York, the new school had not given him any special education services.

Josh was unhappy in school, and falling farther and farther behind. He had a very different attitude toward school than he'd had in Minnesota. The New York teacher dismissed the parents' concerns, saying that Josh was doing fine. But he didn't seem fine to his parents.

Josh hated "resource room," the special small classroom assigned to him for one period a day. It was supposed to give him extra attention to help him catch up with his classwork. However, other students in the resource room had very different needs from Josh. They received most of the special education teacher's attention. Josh said he didn't learn anything in resource room, and felt he had nothing in common with the kids there. For that matter, Josh didn't feel he had anything in common with kids in his regular class either. He felt very alone.

At home, Josh often seemed moody and distracted. He had trouble falling asleep and woke up frequently at night. During the day, he complained often about being tired.

Where to start? When both parent and child have Lyme disease, I usually advise the adult to get help first. I equate it with flight attendants who instruct adult passengers to put on their own oxygen masks before assisting their children. The children will be better off if parents are safe and in control. However, in this case, Josh required immediate attention. He was drowning in school. Despite his best efforts, he could never finish his homework. He could not answer when called on in class. (Was this due to short-term memory loss? Slow processing speed? At this point, I could only speculate.) He was embarrassed by his poor performance, and his mother believed he'd lost all self-confidence. He needed help beyond what his parents, his Lyme doctor, and I could provide. Josh required assessments and advice from a variety of professionals. It was time to expand our team.

The Cornerstone of the Team

The cornerstone of the team is the physician with comprehensive knowledge of Lyme disease. This doctor looks at the overall picture and takes the lead regarding treatment. He or she assesses how the child is doing and what the next step might be. Yet the doctor can't always look at all facets of the problem. Sometimes the expertise of other professionals is needed.

"Dealing with the strictly medical aspects of care is highly challenging in itself," says Dr. Kenneth Liegner, a board-certified internist who has treated Lyme disease for over 25 years. "In straightforward cases, one physician can sometimes 'do it all.' However, involvement of practitioners having specialized expertise that is pertinent to a given child's presenting problems can optimize a child's functioning and recovery."

Josh had an excellent doctor, who had a great deal of compassion for the child and family. He understood how to treat chronic tick-borne diseases, and some of the pitfalls in getting help in school for the child with Lyme. So the choice of physician was a settled matter. However, we also needed the assistance of other professionals, to determine Josh's educational needs and provide vital information about how his brain was functioning. Here are some of the experts we needed for Josh and what their assessments showed:

A Lyme-literate psychiatrist evaluated him for problems with sleep, alertness, cognitive functioning, pain, and irritability—all common with Lyme. The doctor's primary recommendation was sleep medication. He said getting adequate restorative sleep might in fact resolve some of the other problems as well.

A neuropsychologist assessed how Josh's brain was working. This evaluation pointed to specific cognitive deficits that prevented Josh from communicating well. He had problems with short-term memory, organizing his thoughts, and following through. Once his parents learned about this, they realized Josh was not resistant to taking his medication and doing his chores. Rather, he could not remember what he was supposed to do. There were reasons that Josh appeared spacey. This helped his parents find more effective ways to deal with him, and life at home became less stressful for everybody.

A neuro-optometrist found that Josh had double vision, common with Lyme patients. He prescribed prism glasses, specially crafted lenses that keep the eyes working together. The new glasses made it easier for Josh to read his schoolbooks and keep up with class assignments.

Once Tanya saw how much these assessments helped her son, she decided to be evaluated herself. She too was found to need prism glasses. She was also prescribed psycho-active medication, which helped her think more clearly. A neuropsychological evaluation pinpointed her specific cognitive deficits. With this knowledge, she and I devised a variety of coping strategies. Since fatigue made her cognitive issues worse, we planned a schedule that included daily rest times. Given her slow processing speed, we figured out how much time Tanya and Josh needed to prepare for leaving the house each morning. We also came up with a tactic for when she attended school meetings for Josh. When discussions were going too fast, Tanya needed to ask the school staff to repeat whatever she did not understand. It is her right as Josh's mother to understand what is going on in a meeting about her son. If she is comfortable saying so, she can also tell them that she, too, has cognitive problems from Lyme.

Who are some of the other professionals that might be needed on your team?

Neuropsychologist

Neuropsychologists evaluate and treat people with various kinds of nervous system disorders. They examine the relationship between the physical brain and behavior. One of the tools they use is the neuropsychiatric assessment. The website of the Center for Neuropsychology and Counseling in Warrington, PA, defines it this way:

> *A neuropsychological assessment may include tests of the child's intelligence, academic skills, attention and concentration, learning and memory, processing speed, visual spatial perception, language skills, visual motor and fine motor skills, sensory perception, executive functioning (such as planning, organization, initiating and inhibiting behaviors) and emotional functioning. The pediatric neuropsychologist interprets the pattern of results in the context of the child's developmental stage, their current setting, and the child's medical history.*

A thorough neuropsychological evaluation for a child with Lyme disease begins with an interview with the parents. This is followed by about 12 hours of testing the child, generally over three days. It is vital that the neuropsychologist be knowledgeable about Lyme disease. Since many Lyme patients are sensitive to light and sound, she will make sure that the testing environment is appropriate. She'll recognize that the child's ability to function may differ from day to day. She'll be prepared to halt testing if the child becomes overly fatigued. If needed, she'll schedule more days to complete the evaluation. This extensive evaluation, though it may be taxing for the child, is a valuable tool. It quantifies what the child cannot express, particularly when there is a wide spread between the highs in some areas and really low scores in others.

I saw one teenager a few years ago whose parents worried because he was always so quiet. He had been undergoing treatment for Lyme for several years. When Nate walked into my office, he had the sullen demeanor of someone who might be doing drugs or drinking. I couldn't engage him in conversation at all, even when I tried to provoke him. In my view, Nate needed a neuropsychological evaluation as soon as possible. I didn't think depression or behavior problems were behind his apparent unwillingness to communicate. I suspected it was caused by Lyme disease. His parents agreed to take Nate to the practitioner I recommended.

After testing Nate, the neuropsychologist called me. "No wonder you're having trouble engaging him," she said. "Both his expressive and receptive language are severely compromised by Lyme. He doesn't take in what you say, and he has difficulty expressing his thoughts. He simply *can't* communicate." With the parents' blessing, she shared the report with Nate's Lyme doctor. When the doctor realized how extensively Lyme had affected the brain, he put Nate on intravenous antibiotics that were able to cross the blood-brain barrier. IV medications can often resolve such problems more quickly and effectively than oral meds. Because Nate's cognitive impairments had been so thoroughly documented, the insurance company approved the treatment.

Knowing about Nate's language problems also helped me to improve my communications with him. I spoke more slowly (not generally my style), and stuck to one concrete issue at a time. I asked for responses from Nate frequently, to be sure he understood what I had said. His parents and I also informed the school about his communication problems. Thus, accommodations and modifications were put in place to help him.

The treatment had a dramatic effect on Nate. A year later, a follow-up neuropsychological evaluation showed a great deal of improvement. His family also found that he responded when they talked to him, and that he was not as forgetful about his schoolwork and medications.

Lyme-literate Psychiatrist

A psychiatrist who understands how Lyme disease affects the brain can help the child with a host of problems. According to Dr. Robert Bransfield, many late-stage pediatric symptoms are neuropsychiatric and can be demonstrated objectively with mental status evaluations, psychiatric testing, and brain imagery. He says that three of the biggest issues a child with Lyme may face are non-restorative sleep, fatigue, and cognitive impairments. "Treatments that increase Delta sleep and normalize circadian rhythm help these symptoms."

Bransfield notes that children sometimes need traditional psychotropic medications for anxiety, depression, or psychosis. Other strategies might include further treatment to improve cognitive function, stress reduction, pain management, diet and exercise.

In my practice, I find that addressing sleep is the most pressing issue for many Lyme patients. Lack of restorative sleep can increase pain and make it harder for the child to think, focus, and concentrate. In fact, I rarely see a Lyme patient who can get restorative sleep without the help of medication, although some are helped with naturopathic remedies. I often find that many of my clients' symptoms improve dramatically when their psychiatrists address sleep issues first.

However, psychiatrists who are not familiar with tick-borne illness may prescribe medication that is not targeted toward the Lyme patient's most pressing problem. The more expansive role of psychopharmacology for Lyme patients is overlooked. I therefore only make referrals to psychiatrists who are knowledgeable about Lyme disease. It is important to note that my role is not to diagnose or determine which psychotropic medications should be prescribed. That is up to the psychiatrist. But I can help parents hone in on the most important items to discuss with their doctor.

In preparing a child and parents for the appointment with the psychiatrist, I discuss the importance of identifying which symptoms make it hard for the patient to function on a daily basis. In addition to sleep, I ask about attention, concentration, impulsivity, pain, anxiety, OCD, and rage. If the child exhibits any high-risk behaviors, it's essential to discuss that with the doctor, as well. The child must be protected from harming himself or others, even as the Lyme is being treated.

As we talk about what else the child and parents would like to see improve, I begin to assess what may be triggering these symptoms. For example, if a child is anxious and resists going to school, I need to know why. Is he being bullied? (Many years ago, an 11-year-old client of mine had a facial tic brought on by Lyme. He was badly beaten by a school bully because he "wouldn't stop twitching.") Can he do his schoolwork? What's the hardest thing about the work itself? What accommodations does he need to feel safe and to function well in the school setting? If the child is still anxious after these supports are in place, I do suggest that the parents ask the psychiatrist about medication. I also recommend that the parents look into yoga, meditation, or mindfulness training for their child, which can help reduce anxiety.

Focus and concentration are often significant issues, so those might be on my list. Chronic pain may need to be addressed by medication that is safe for children. The parents, the child, and I join in making the list of symptoms that interfere with the child's ability to function. Then, when they see the psychiatrist, they can zero in on the most important issues.

Licensed Clinical Social Worker

A psychosocial assessment evaluates a person's mental health, social wellbeing, and how he functions in the community. It is generally done by a social worker, who looks at family history, diagnosed physical or mental illness, and other factors. It takes into account the physical health of the client, as well as her perception of self and ability to function. It is used to create a comprehensive picture of the client and helps in developing goals. The social worker who conducts the psychosocial assessment needs to recognize that Lyme symptoms are so unpredictable, and the illness is so poorly understood, that venturing out into the community can be very difficult. This is not generally because of any mental illness on the part of the Lyme disease patient or any family dysfunction. It is part of the illness and society's response to Lyme patients and their families.

Schools may request psychosocial assessments of children with Lyme disease to aid in education planning. It can be a useful tool when parents are advocating for the child in school. It may also be important in contentious divorces, in which one parent may claim that the other is mentally ill. In the juvenile justice system, a psychosocial evaluation can provide a valuable assessment of how the child and family function, as well.

However, if the professional doing the assessment doesn't understand tick-borne disease, the conclusions, definition of the problem, and strategies for moving forward will be flawed. These inaccurate results might be used against the child and family—in school, and even with the courts. They may lead the school to take actions that involve social services or the juvenile justice system. In contrast, an accurate psychosocial assessment can be a family's saving grace. It can bring valuable information before school teams, social service agencies, and even family courts. Parents would do well to find a Lyme-literate social worker for this assessment.

Neuro-Optometrist/Neuro-Ophthalmologist

These professionals look at neurological causes of vision problems. Lyme disease can disrupt a child's ability to read and otherwise process information. There may be problems with balance, dizziness, headaches, glare sensitivity, panic attacks, and reduced sight. Many of these symptoms can be treated by various vision therapies, including the use of prism eyeglasses. See appendix for more information.

Why Further Evaluations Might Be Needed

The neuropsychologist may recommend other assessments, depending on the testing results and clinical observations. For instance, if your child has a hard time telling the difference between similar-sounding words, this might indicate an auditory processing disorder that should be followed up by an audiologist. Problems with expressive and receptive language (speaking and understanding) might require a speech-language pathologist. Lack of fine motor coordination, which may show up as difficulty tying shoes or using scissors, should be evaluated by an occupational therapist. Reports from these experts can document what educational supports the child needs to succeed in the classroom.

Depending on how complicated your child's case is, there may also be a need to consult medical specialists, such as cardiologists, neurologists, endocrinologists, or immunologists. Ideally, your Lyme doctor would be able to refer to you to someone with an understanding of Lyme disease. Unfortunately, that's not always possible. You may have to deal with a specialist who adheres to the Infectious Diseases Society of America's (IDSA) restricted views about Lyme disease treatment. If so, I recommend that you prepare carefully for such visits, providing documentation for all of your child's symptoms.

nine

Educating Your Child
With Lyme Disease

Sandy:

CAITLIN WAS AN EIGHTH GRADER who loved everything about school. She participated eagerly in class, her hand shooting up as soon as the teacher asked a question. She found learning easy, had no problems finishing her homework, and earned good grades. She had a lot of friends, and enjoyed seeing them both in and out of school.

Things changed in ninth grade, though the differences were subtle at first. Homework took longer. She complained of frequent headaches and stomach aches. At night, she'd toss and turn for hours and then be exhausted in the morning. Although her parents took her to different doctors, no one could determine what was wrong. Finally, in November of tenth grade, Caitlyn was diagnosed with Lyme disease. She'd probably contracted it the summer before her freshman year.

Lyme disease can drastically impact a child's education. One of the biggest problems involves sleep—both too much and too little.

Some children may sleep many more hours than is common for others their age. But from what I have seen, for most young Lyme patients it is just the opposite. They cannot get enough sleep and what little they get is of poor quality. Some children completely reverse their circadian rhythms. They stay awake all night and sleep during the day. Those around them may see this as a behavior problem and assume the child is staying awake to defy the parent. But for the great majority of children with Lyme, the sleep problems are, in fact, caused by the disease.

Such sleep problems can contribute to profound fatigue. Blogger Jennifer Crystal, who writes extensively about the experience of having Lyme disease, describes it this way:

> *The fatigue of tick-borne diseases...is a crippling flu-like exhaustion, one that leaves muscles not sore but literally unable to function; one that makes the body feel shackled to the bed; one that makes the effort of lifting one's head off the pillow seem like a Herculean feat. There were times, at my lowest point of illness, when I ...felt too tired to breathe.*

Another symptom that interferes with education is pain. Children with Lyme may have migraine-like headaches, joint pain or gastrointestinal disturbances. One of my young clients would spend up to two hours in the bathroom at a stretch, crying in agony, as her mother tried to comfort her. This unpredictable symptom made it impossible for this child to attend school. She needed homebound instruction until, with proper medical treatment, this problem cleared up.

Sensitivity to light and sound makes school intolerable for some students with Lyme. The noise of children in the halls and cafeteria may be overwhelming. For some, even the sound of a pencil scratching on a paper is too much. Fluorescent lighting in the classroom can cause burning eyes, blurred vision, or severe headaches. Furthermore, children whose brains have been affected by Lyme disease may find it extremely hard to process information and organize their time. They may have problems involving short-term memory and word-finding.

In my practice, I have not met a child with Lyme who wanted to get out of going to school when healthy enough to do so. The children I see want to attend school and to connect with their peers. Before getting sick, some had been active in sports, music, or drama. Even the quiet or shy children had found their circle of friends and their place in school.

The picture changes when Lyme symptoms emerge. (See Berenbaum Screening Protocol in Appendix D.) At first, there might be subtle backsliding, as school attendance and performance gradually decline. After the child has been diagnosed, the parents may realize that problems at school are due to the disease and not her failure to try her best. Unfortunately, many schools do not understand the link between the illness and academic performance. It can be useful to help educate district personnel about Lyme disease, to minimize the level of misunderstanding between the school and the family.

Here are some of the school-related problems that children with Lyme may experience:

- Attendance—Sometimes the child is too ill to be in class. Other times, there are medical appointments that cannot be scheduled after school. Some schools have firm attendance and lateness policies that don't make allowances for such circumstances. For children with a documented medical need to be out of school, it is important to establish a 504 plan or an Individualized Education Program (IEP) that includes a waiver of the attendance and tardiness policies. (See below for discussion of 504s and IEPs.)

- Length of school day—The regular academic day is too long for many children with Lyme. Some schools may agree to a shortened day, but want the child to start early in the morning when the other students arrive. That rarely works for students with the sleep problems that are typical of Lyme. They often wake up later and take longer to get ready. A shortened day, starting late, may help them stay in school and better absorb the material.
- Bathroom access—Children with gastrointestinal symptoms must be free to go to the bathroom as needed. They should not have to ask the teacher's permission first. This meets a physical need and avoids embarrassing the student. Some schools will easily provide this kind of support for children who need it. They may even allow the child to use the bathroom in the nurse's office to avoid the more public student facilities.
- Access to a quiet room—Students suffering from sensory overload or headaches need a chance to escape to a quiet place. This might be the nurse's office or a room off of the teacher's lounge. Taking a break like this may protect the rest of the day, and avoid the need for the child to leave school early or go on homebound instruction.

No two cases of Lyme are exactly alike, with identical symptoms and challenges. There is no blueprint for educating a child with Lyme disease. Complex problems call for complex solutions.

Public schools are charged with providing an education for every child, even those with a medical illness. Ideally, teachers and parents will collaborate in figuring out the best way to meet a child's needs. To facilitate this, parents must be ready to discuss the nature of the illness, focusing on what their child needs in school. The school will probably ask for documentation, starting with a letter from the treating physician. This should provide the diagnosis, the doctor's assessment of the student's limitations, and a list of her medications.

In my view, additional medical information, such as the results of blood tests, should remain private. If school officials want to see medical records or evaluations, ask them to put their request in writing. You should also ask them to designate what educational purpose having that information will serve. You can pass that written request along to your doctor, who can also respond in writing.

Many students with chronic Lyme disease need specific assistance in the classroom. Sometimes modest adjustments can make a world of difference. A letter from the doctor can define the child's symptoms and suggest ways to handle them at school. Some examples are:

- "Susie's medications require her to stay well hydrated. It would be helpful for her to carry a water bottle and drink from it as needed throughout the day."
- "Her medications can lead to an urgent need to use the bathroom. She should not have to wait for the teacher to grant permission each time."
- "Due to Susie's profound fatigue and joint pain, she is unable to take physical education at this time."
- "Susie has severe joint pains, difficulty with sleep, and profound fatigue. This may impact her ability to attend school regularly or remain in school for a full day."

If a student uses a wheelchair or has seizures in class, teachers may readily grasp the severity of the illness. But many students with Lyme don't look sick. Thus, school staff may not appreciate how ill these children actually are, and may fail to grasp why the student needs special consideration. This may strain the relationship between the school and the parents. However, I don't presume that the relationship between parents and school will always be contentious. Instead, I work with the parents to help school authorities have a better understanding of the child's situation.

As with everything else I do, I seek to solve problems. At first, we make sure that the child's illness has been properly documented for the school. Furthermore, I offer school officials an opportunity to learn more about Lyme disease. When I attend meetings, I often bring along informative articles to give the staff. Sometimes this really makes a difference. Educators with a better understanding of how Lyme impacts schooling may be more willing to find ways to help the student. Thus, the process of collaboration is underway.

IEPs and 504 Plans—Legal Entitlements for Children With Disabilities

Many students with chronic Lyme disease may need more than informal supports in the classroom. If they meet the criteria to be designated as "disabled," their educational rights are defined under two specific bodies of law. Under these laws, the parents and school work together to create a plan for the child's education.

Section 504 of the Rehabilitation Act of 1973 extends civil rights to people with disabilities. That law, referred as the **504 plan**, says that no one with a disability can be excluded from federally funded programs, including public schooling. The goal is to "level the playing field" for children who have disabilities identified under the law. According to the website of the U.S. Office of Civil Rights:

A medical diagnosis of an illness does not automatically mean a student can receive services under Section 504. The illness must cause a substantial limitation on the student's ability to learn or another major life activity. For example, a student who has a physical or mental impairment would not be considered a student in need of services under Section 504 if the impairment does not in any way limit the student's ability to learn or other major life activity, or only results in some minor limitation in that regard.

A written 504 plan is a legal document that the teachers are expected to follow. It should specify which "accommodations and modifications" the child needs. For example, if his processing speed is slow, he may need extra time to complete assignments and examinations. If he is sensitive to sound and easily distracted, he may need a quiet place to take tests. These are common classroom accommodations that can be put into 504 plans.

A child who has problems with "word finding," an inability to recall words, would have difficulty with fill-in-the-blanks tests. In this case, he could be given a list of words, called a "word bank," instead of having to fill in the blanks from memory. Someone with profound fatigue or slow processing speed could have shortened writing assignments. The child's grade should not suffer because he's writing a shorter paper. Some schools write into the 504 plan "graded on work completed." This is for children who are so fatigued and physically impaired that it is impossible to predict how much work can be completed every day or every week.

An **Individualized Educational Plan (IEP)** addresses the need for specialized instruction or remediation for a child who has a disability identified under the Individuals with Disabilities Education Act (IDEA). This body of law designates the specific process needed to determine eligibility for special education classification and to develop the IEP. The goal is to provide a "free and appropriate public education" (FAPE) for a child who is classified. A child who does not need specialized instruction, remediation, or services only available to special education students, does not qualify for an IEP.

Generally, getting a 504 plan is less complicated and can be done more quickly than going through the IEP process. Since time is of the essence when a child is quickly falling behind in school, most parents start with the 504 plan. Then if the parents think their child needs services not covered by the 504, they will pursue an IEP.

Parents must begin the IEP process by sending a written request for a comprehensive evaluation of their child to the school's director of special education. They should state that they have reason to believe their child has a disability and that they are concerned that the student's educational needs are not being met without an IEP. This begins the process of determining whether a child meets the criteria for classification.

One classification that I suggest parents be wary of is emotionally disturbed (ED). It's not an appropriate label for most children with Lyme disease. If anxiety, depressed mood, and behavior problems (such as rages) were not present before the child became ill, then these are in all likelihood symptoms of Lyme disease. This is not an "emotional disturbance," and I suggest that parents not agree to this label. It might prompt the school to place the student in a program that is unsuitable for someone who is medically ill. Educational planning may go in an entirely different direction than is beneficial for a child with Lyme, using instruments and strategies that won't help, and may in fact be counterproductive.

Several classifications are appropriate and accurate for many students with Lyme disease. Most of these students meet the criteria for other health impaired (OHI). Some with severe brain symptoms meet the educational classification of traumatic brain injury (TBI). (Note: the definition of TBI for special education may be different from the medical definition of TBI. It requires specific documentation designated under state education law.) Children with Lyme may also fit the "learning disabled" classification.

The most common document to support a Special Education classification for children with Lyme disease is the neuropsychological evaluation. (This is discussed in Chapter Eight). A single-photon emission computed tomography (SPECT) brain scan, showing problems with blood flow in the brain, may also be accepted by the school for TBI classification.

Some children may already have a special education classification for an issue unrelated to Lyme disease. One example is speech/language impairment. Perhaps the student had exhibited language problems even before the Lyme diagnosis. Rather than starting the process anew, it's less complicated to get additional services put into the existing IEP. Maintaining the original classification keeps the IEP in place, in case it is still needed after Lyme-related symptoms have resolved.

When I met Sammy, he was 9 years old and in fourth grade. A talkative child, he readily told me about his many interests. He was very bright, identifying the trees outside my office window and teaching me about their growth patterns. An only child, he loved playing with his cousins and was not depressed or socially isolated. He told me he wanted to become an architect and design buildings. However, when I asked him if he liked to build with Legos, his face clouded up. He said he couldn't do Legos.

As it turned out, Sammy had a special education classification because of his very poor fine motor coordination. This is the set of movements that allow actions, such as picking up a Lego or writing with a pencil or pen. Sammy had been in treatment for Lyme disease for about four years, having had it for most of his young life. Although he was highly intelligent, it took him much longer to do his work than his classmates. For instance, he needed ten hours to complete a written assignment that his classmates finished in about two hours. Even though he tried hard, he was falling further and further behind in school and couldn't catch up. He became more and more frustrated.

I referred Sammy for a neuropsychological evaluation, which confirmed my suspicions. He needed more than the occupational therapy provided in his current IEP. The neuropsychologist recommended that Sammy use assistive technology, such as a computer keyboard, iPad, or dictation software. This would allow him to work more quickly and easily than writing by hand. Significant problems with processing speed, word finding, and other cognitive issues called for additional modifications and accommodations as well. The neuropsychological evaluation gave us documentation to advocate for the services Sammy needed.

I met Melanie when she was 10 years old and in fifth grade. Before Lyme, she had been a physically active child, diagnosed with a speech delay at age 2. She received speech-language services from age 2 to 3. By age 8, she was identified in the school as having problems with both expressive and receptive language. She met the criteria for a speech/language classification. By fourth grade, she had an IEP, providing her with the services of a speech pathologist. Also in fourth grade, she started missing school due to episodes of severe abdominal pain and insomnia. Her parents took her to many doctors, who failed to determine what was wrong. Eventually, she was diagnosed with Lyme disease and began treatment. When I met her, she was on homebound instruction.

Her family came to me because the situation with the school district had become contentious. The person in charge of students on homebound instruction refused to accept the doctor's letter. Instead, he pressured the parents to send Melanie back to school. The parents followed their Lyme doctor's recommendation to keep the girl home. Then, the district filed allegations of "educational neglect" with Child Protective Services. The district charged the parents with endangering their daughter's welfare by keeping her out of school.

School officials said Melanie suffered from an "emotional illness," perhaps school phobia, separation anxiety, or an anxiety disorder. They pushed to have her back in class. This was highly inappropriate. Anxieties and phobias are diagnoses of mental illness. School personnel aren't qualified to diagnose students. Yet, that's what they appeared to be doing with Melanie. Furthermore, if the school had reason to believe Melanie had an emotional illness, they should have been trying to get her special services, not taking them away from her.

As a licensed clinical social worker and her therapist, I wrote a report to her school. My assessment of Melanie and her family indicated that she did not appear to suffer from a mental illness. Her symptoms were typical of children with chronic tick-borne disease. I referred Melanie to a Lyme-literate psychiatrist, who also found Melanie's symptoms to be consistent with tick-borne disease. He found no phobia, anxiety, or other mental illness. At my suggestion, Melanie also had a neuropsychological evaluation. It showed that she had deficits often seen in students with Lyme disease. The neuropsychologist wrote, "It is important to keep in mind that Melanie is always functioning against a background of pain, sensory sensitivity, and auditory processing difficulty."

However, the school continued to deny that Lyme was the cause of any of Melanie's problems. Her family worried that another allegation of neglect would be filed with CPS. Melanie's parents retained an attorney and a Lyme-knowledgeable education advocate. I also attended IEP meetings with the parents, as a Lyme expert and as the child's and family's psychotherapist. The district continued to demand that Melanie come back in school, despite the well-documented findings of her physician and other professionals.

Eventually, the family filed a complaint with the state's Department of Education. It charged that the person overseeing homebound instruction had violated Melanie's right to medical privacy by contacting her doctor without signed consent from her parents. The family won its case. The ruling required that the school employee in question have nothing more do with Melanie's educational planning. CPS dropped all charges. Homebound instruction continued, and Melanie obtained the supports she needed to continue her education.

A few lessons from Melanie's story:

- It is possible to prevail through the appeals process, even with an uncooperative school district.

- When the school is not open to collaboration, it is important to build an effective team of professionals who know about Lyme disease. This certainly would include your child's Lyme doctor. Others on the team may be a psychotherapist, an education advocate, a psychiatrist, a neuropsychologist, and possibly an education attorney.

- Parents who want to appeal the school's decision need to be ready to build a case. This will involve researching the legal issues, extensively documenting, and preparing carefully for all meetings with the school. Hiring an education advocate can help. Education advocates are trained in how to deal with schools effectively. However, it is vital that the advocate be Lyme-literate, or at least open to learning about the disease.

- Consent is an important concept to understand. It must be voluntary. If parents are uncomfortable with anything the school proposes, they should not consent to it. For instance, you can refuse to allow the school to talk to your child's doctor without your being present. You can refuse to consent to the doctor releasing any information that is not necessary for education planning for your child.

I can't emphasize enough how important it is to document the child's disability for school officials. Qualified professionals must support the designation of the disability and determine the need for special services. If the school advises you that they are attributing the child's school issues to a psychiatric disorder or family dysfunction, it is valuable to address that, either in the doctor's letter, or in documentation from a mental health practitioner the child is seeing.

Education Advocate

As mentioned above, some parents find it helpful to engage the services of an education advocate. An advocate understands special education law, on both the federal and state levels. Usually, advocates have special training in this field. Many belong to the Council of Parent Attorney and Advocates (COPAA). Education advocates guide parents through the complicated process of obtaining special school services for their child. They may also attend school meetings with the parents. It is vital that the education advocate understand the unique challenges of Lyme disease.

Education Attorneys

Families who believe they have run into a brick wall in their efforts to meet their child's educational needs may feel compelled to hire an attorney. If so, it is essential to find one who specializes in education law. This attorney should also understand the roadblocks specific to families with Lyme disease. Once the parents have hired an attorney, the school usually brings its own attorney to the school meetings. Unfortunately, at that point the process may become adversarial rather than collaborative. To find education advocates or attorneys who specialize in education law, check out the COPAA website (www.copaa.org).

Homebound Instruction

When a student is too ill to attend regular school, the district is obligated to provide for his education another way. Sometimes this is called "homebound instruction," "home/hospital instruction," or "medical independent study." The goal is to help students keep up their studies, so they can return to school without falling too far behind. Typically, these programs send a teacher or tutor to the child's home for an hour or two, several times per week. (This is different from "homeschooling," discussed later in this chapter.)

There are various reasons why students with Lyme may need homebound instruction. Physical disability or pain may make it difficult or impossible to even leave the house. They may be too fatigued to function in the classroom, even for part of the day. Their immune systems may be too weak to withstand being exposed to infections that other students might carry.

Yet, even with homebound instruction, there may be problems. School administrators expect students to "show up for school" on schedule, even if it happens in the family's living room. But strict timetables often don't work for children with Lyme disease. Symptom flares and lack of sleep may make it impossible for them to participate at their assigned hour. However, parents who postpone too many sessions may run into trouble with school officials. Ideally, homebound instruction would be planned to meet the child's needs. For many, the best time would be in the late afternoon. However, sometimes the school has a different idea about when homebound instruction should take place. Parents need to be familiar with the federal and state rules regarding homebound instruction. Helpful information may be found on copaa.org or wrightslaw.com.

Some states limit homebound instruction to a few months. If a student can't return to the regular classroom within that time, schools may offer different kinds of independent study programs. Unfortunately, the available options may not be suitable for a particular child's medical needs. Sometimes the issues involved are so complex that parents may want the services of an education advocate or attorney to sort things out and make sure their child's needs are being appropriately met.

I have seen tremendous success in educating children who are too ill to attend regular classes. Timothy, an 18-year-old high school senior, had been a good student and a gifted athlete before he contracted Lyme disease. Not diagnosed early, the Lyme became chronic. Timothy had an excellent doctor and was making progress, but the road to recovery was long and slow. Tim hated that he could no longer compete in athletics, a large part of his identity. He was devastated when he couldn't go to school. He didn't know how he could even graduate from high school, let alone prepare for college.

Fortunately, Tim's school district had a good system in place for students needing homebound instruction. He was put on a 504 plan that gave him a reduced workload, with no penalty for late assignments and extra time for testing. For some subjects, he could answer questions orally rather than in writing. He worked diligently with his tutors, although sometimes severe symptoms forced him to cancel a session. Through homebound instruction, Tim graduated from high school and went on to college.

Specialized Public School Programs

Some school districts offer alternative high school programs for students who don't do well in the traditional classroom. These "last chance" options are often geared to at-risk youth with severe behavior problems and are not designed for students with serious medical conditions. They are not usually a good fit for a child with Lyme disease.

Depending on where you live, your district may offer something that works better for your child. In California, for instance, many districts offer independent study programs in which a child is guided by a teacher but does not take classes with other students. This is different from homebound instruction. Usually, the student has a weekly session with the teacher and works independently the rest of the time. This can be a good choice for students capable of studying on their own, though it is not a suitable choice for everyone.

Alternatives to Public Education

Private school may be a viable option for some families who can afford it. Classes tend to be smaller, and parents may see the quality of instruction as better. Some private schools are specifically designed to educate students with learning disabilities, and some students with Lyme-related cognitive problems might do well at them. However, there are no mandated 504 plans or IEPs, since these bodies of law only apply to institutions that receive public funds. In addition, private schools are generally not equipped to provide special services for disabled children.

Homeschooling—with the child not enrolled in school at all—is another option. The parents and child develop a homeschooling plan that complies with requirements of the state in which they live. The parent takes responsibility for making sure the plan is carried out.

There are different ways of homeschooling. Some families sign up for a specific boxed (or online) curriculum. This may come with textbooks, a schedule of what to study when, and a method for keeping records and assigning grades. The other end of the spectrum is what some people call "unschooling." This uses no formal schedules or texts, and instead allows children to follow their interests. Other models lie somewhere in between. According to the website homeschooling.com:

'Relaxed' *or* **'eclectic'** *homeschooling is the method used most often by homeschoolers. Basically, eclectic homeschoolers use a little of this and a little of that, using workbooks for math, reading, and spelling, and taking an 'unschooling' approach for the other subjects.*

Such a relaxed system allows for the flexibility a chronically ill child needs. You may follow general curriculum guidelines, yet tailor your approach to the individual child.

Homeschooling is legal throughout the United States, though regulations vary from state-to-state. According the website ResponsibleHomeschooling.org:

> *Most states require parents to notify state or local education officials of their intent to homeschool, and half of all states have some form of assessment requirement. Most states have days of instruction or subject requirements and a smaller number of states have parent qualification and bookkeeping requirements. Some states require none of the above.*

It is essential that you learn the homeschooling regulations for your state. Even if you are within your legal rights to homeschool your child, local school authorities may view it differently. The Home School Legal Defense Association (HSLDA) advocates for homeschooling families. The organization's website recounts the following story about parents whose daughter had Lyme disease:

> *The family had been investigated previously, several times, because of relatives who disagreed with the family's choice to homeschool. The most recent referral, however, was made by a medical provider who wanted the girl in school for "social reasons" and who further accused the mother of "pathologizing" her daughter with too many doctor visits. Although the girl was being treated by a Lyme specialist and had been positively diagnosed with Lyme, social workers continued to conduct a longer term "family assessment," creating increased stress on the family.*

The HSLDA intervened on the family's behalf, and charges were eventually dropped.

Online learning is becoming more widely available. Some programs may be accessed through your own school district, while others may fall under the homeschooling model. Online programs vary widely. It is important to consider the needs of the specific student. For instance, some online programs require that the work be completed within a defined time frame. This may not be a good choice for a student who is ill. An open-ended program that allows a student to work at his own pace may be a better fit.

College Courses for High School Credit

In some areas, high school students can attend "dual" or "concurrent" classes at a local community college, earning both high school and college credits for the same course. This can be a good choice for some chronically ill students, since college classes typically offer flexible scheduling. Thus, a student can attend during his most productive time of day. Also, colleges draw students from a broader area, so there may not be the clique atmosphere that exists in many high schools. Some students who have been away from school find the "re-entry" process easier at a community college. Usually, high school students must be juniors or seniors to enroll in dual-credit college classes. They must also meet the college's prerequisite requirements for any individual course.

Students who do not complete high school may be eligible to get a high school equivalency certificate. Requirements vary by state, but generally involve passing a test in various subject matters. Before 2014, all states used a standard General Education Development (GED) test. In 2014, the landscape changed considerably. The company that makes the GED test offered a revised, computer-based version. Also, two new testing companies entered the picture. Some states changed their requirements and now offer one, two, or all three of these options.

- GED—The new GED exam measures proficiency in four subject areas: reasoning through language arts, mathematical reasoning, science, and social studies. Testing is done by computer.

- TASC—The Test Assessing Secondary Completion is available via computer and on paper. It tests science, math, social studies, reading, and writing.

- **HiSET**—The High School Equivalency Test assesses science, math, social studies, reading, and writing. It is available on either computer or paper.

All three testing companies say they offer accommodations as needed to disabled students, which might include a separate testing room, more time, or extra breaks. All such requests must be handled in advance of the testing day. Be prepared to document the student's need for the requested service.

Obtaining a high school equivalency certificate opens the way for the student to move on to college or the workplace. I have had several clients who pursued that route. Now in college, some have told me that they were pleased that they had made that choice.

Despite all of these options, some children with Lyme are unable to do any schoolwork at all. Some school districts understand, once they've reviewed the documentation from the various professionals. That's not the case with others. Parents may justifiably worry that the school district might report them for educational neglect. I recommend that parents in this situation consult an education advocate and/or education attorney. Comprehensive documentation of their child's health status and needs is essential.

Dorothy:

My daughter missed most of eighth grade. We tried the home/hospital program, in which the school district sent a teacher to our house. However, Rachel's pain, fatigue, and memory problems made it impossible for her to do school work. Occasionally, she enjoyed listening to me read aloud from one of her books. Then, perhaps an hour later, she would not remember that I'd read anything to her at all.

Our doctor wrote a letter explaining this. Yet, the school district pressured me to bring her back to school, use the home teacher, or enroll her in independent study. They didn't accept that she was too ill to do any schooling at all. They seemed to think I *wanted* my child to fall behind. They told me about a local boy who had graduated at the top of his class, despite having chemotherapy during his senior year. They often repeated, "and he had *cancer*." Their message seemed to be, "He was worse off than your daughter, yet he still went to school."

By the beginning of ninth grade, Rachel's cognitive abilities were improving. Though still in pain and still in the wheelchair, she wanted to return to school. She attended one class a day—seventh period Spanish. I'd push her wheelchair over to the junior high school and bring her home an hour later. I don't think she particularly cared about learning Spanish. However, she loved being in class with other kids, especially one girl who became a close friend. Yet, I doubt that the teacher or anyone else knew how much attending that Spanish class sapped Rachel's energy.

As her treatment for Lyme continued, various symptoms showed improvement. By the second semester of ninth grade, she wanted to try a little more academic work. While she continued to take Spanish in school, we tried an online class at home. We chose Brigham Young University's online high school program for its flexibility. Rachel could start a class at any time, move at her own pace, and have up to a year to complete it.

The experiment was a success. By the end of the school year, she had completed two semester-long online classes, earning an A in English and a B in algebra. Although I oversaw her English assignments, algebra was out of my league. So, we hired a college student—a pleasant young woman who was majoring in math—as a tutor. They used the online algebra program as their text and worked at a pace that Rachel could handle. They seemed to enjoy themselves quite a bit, and Rachel always looked forward to the twice-weekly sessions.

About this time, Rachel also started taking a class in American Sign Language (ASL) offered at a church in our town. She had become fascinated with sign language after watching *The Miracle Worker*, about the life of Helen Keller. The class met once a week for an hour and involved no homework. It was just a diverse group of people who wanted to learn ASL. She loved it.

So, near the end of ninth grade, I wasn't worried when a counselor from the junior high asked to meet with me to discuss Rachel's plans for tenth grade. I was thrilled with the headway my daughter was making. Previously, she'd been unable to retain information from even a single paragraph. Now, she could hold her own while studying Spanish, English, algebra, and sign language. She had also recently taught herself to produce small videos and had learned to crochet. She was still in pain, still needed a wheelchair, and still struggled with fatigue and other symptoms. But as her health slowly improved, her mind was clearing. Working in small bites—an hour here and there, with plenty of rest in between—allowed her to make steady progress. Furthermore, both video editing and crocheting were artistic outlets that brought her pleasure. I saw her inner spirit waking up after lying dormant for so long. Hope had returned to our house!

Regrettably, that's not how the school district saw it, at all. I walked into that meeting expecting to see a school guidance counselor. Instead, I was met with a committee of people, including a district administrator who seemed very unhappy with me. She said it had recently come to her attention that Rachel was attending only one class at the junior high. She said this violated district policy and was grounds for charges of truancy. Since the school year was almost over, she'd let it go for now. However, she warned me, high school would be a different story, and we shouldn't expect to "get away with anything."

I tried to explain about Rachel's health problems and offered a copy of our doctor's letter. The administrator didn't want to hear it. When I told the committee about Rachel's progress in English and algebra, a counselor interrupted me to say, "You can't honestly believe that an online class is as good as sitting in school with a trained teacher!" I was flabbergasted. They acted as if my only goal was to keep my daughter out of school, and as if their only goal was to prevent me from doing so. The conversation didn't seem to be about how to meet my daughter's medical and educational needs at all.

I explained to the committee that because Rachel's ability to do schoolwork was improving, she hoped to take two classes at the high school the following year—drama and English. The faces around the table stared at me like I was an alien with antennae sticking out of my head. Not possible, they said. In order to take two classes at the high school, she would need to take an additional four classes through the district's independent study program. (These were not online classes. The program involved meeting with a teacher once a week and working out of the textbook on her own the rest of the time.)

Six classes? That was a big leap. Hadn't anything I'd said sunk in? Along with all of her other symptoms, at one point Rachel had been so cognitively impaired she couldn't read and understand a paragraph. As her treatment had kicked in, there had been some improvement, but she was by no means where she needed to be to take on a full schedule. While cheering her progress, our doctor strongly cautioned us against having her take on too much at once. He said he'd seen too many kids with Lyme begin to improve, return to fulltime schooling, and then have a serious relapse. Following his guidance, our plan was to continue slowly ramping up her activity, one baby step at a time.

Two classes at the high school might not have seemed like much to this committee. But it would double Rachel's current academic schedule. If she could manage that, we might slowly increase her workload. Of course we wanted her back in school. However, we did not want to set her up for academic failure or for a medical relapse. That's why we wanted to start with only those two classes.

Not possible, the administrator insisted. Rachel's choices were these:

- attend high school full time (which our doctor said was out of the question, and we agreed);
- enroll in the independent study program full time (which wouldn't allow her to take drama or see friends at school and would be too rigorous an academic load);
- or take two classes at the high school, along with four in the independent study program (again, too heavy a schedule).

Several times during the meeting I asked, "Why are those our only choices?" Each time, I heard the same puzzling reply. "It's much better for your daughter this way."

Huh?

About a week later, I happened to speak to a mother who had several special-needs children attending local schools. Although her family's circumstances were different from ours, she knew a lot about how the educational system worked. After hearing my story, she said, "Funding."

"What?"

"That's how funding works. If your daughter only attended one class this past year, the district didn't get any money for her from the state. If they let her attend just two classes at the high school next year, they still won't get any money. A student must be enrolled in a certain number of classes in order for the school district to receive funding."

"What if she isn't capable of meeting that minimum?"

The mother shrugged. "Doesn't matter."

⌘

Rachel started tenth grade by enrolling in drama and English at the high school, along with the four easiest classes we could find in the independent study program's schedule. I wasn't sure she could pull it off, but I honored her desire to try.

At first, Rachel assumed she'd enjoy her regular high school classes more than independent study. Ironically, the opposite happened. Because independent study could be tailored to her own needs, it worked out better than the high school's one-size-fits-all approach. By eleventh grade, even though Rachel no longer needed a wheelchair, she enrolled full time in this alternative program and stayed there until graduation. Three wonderful teachers helped her design a curriculum that met her personal needs and interests.

In her junior year, Rachel also took American Sign Language classes at community college, earning both high school and college credits. She continued with ASL her senior year, and also volunteered weekly in a classroom for deaf and hard-of-hearing children. This valuable "real world" experience led to her decision to pursue a career focused on deaf education. Yet, her experience with ASL paid off more immediately, as well.

Although Lyme treatment had cleared up some of her cognitive deficits by this point, Rachel still had problem areas. For instance, she might read a book and write a report on it. Then, by the following week, she'd be unable to remember much about either the book or what she had written. She also found it virtually impossible to memorize facts she needed to know for tests. No matter how much she studied, she couldn't retain the information.

One day, faced with a list of historic events she was going to be tested on, she decided to experiment. Rachel translated the terms into sign language and memorized them that way. She found she could remember the material easily and did well on the test. Incorporating sign language like this helped her successfully complete high school. Later, we found out that some educators promote the use of sign language in the general classroom. According to the website schoolhealth.com,

Research has shown that pairing signs with English helps learners formulate mental pictures. This multi-modal experience can help create new pathways in the brain for storage and retrieval. This helps students remember and recall sight words and spelling words.

LessonPlanet, a website for teachers, calls sign language "a beneficial teaching tool that promotes cognitive functioning." Rachel discovered that by herself.

Here's my message to parents of children with Lyme. Find the educational option that works best for your child's situation. Maybe it will be a program offered by your school district, or maybe not. The best choice will vary from person to person and may change at different times for the same child.

Recognize the distinction between schooling and education. Sometimes children are too sick for schooling, but they can still learn. Help your children make discoveries that capture their imaginations, perhaps via music, art, or computers. These can be tried in small doses, as the child feels up to it. Sometimes taking part in an activity in a limited way—like my daughter's initial foray into sign language—paves the way for deeper exploration later on.

ten

After High School

Dorothy:

COMPLETING HIGH SCHOOL is a significant accomplishment for any student with chronic Lyme. For many, it has required a lot of strategizing, planning, and sheer effort. What happens next will depend upon the health status, capabilities, and interests of your student. It's important for you and your son or daughter to examine options carefully.

Some young people know what they want to pursue next and just need to figure out how best to do it. For others, their vision of the future is less clear. (Even those with no health problems can fall into that category.) Young adulthood can be a time of uncertainty and exploration. As a parent, a good place to start this conversation is by discussing your child's passions and interests. How does she imagine her life might look in the future?

Some young people may want to start college right away. Others may want to get a job. Still others may feel that finishing high school took every ounce of effort they could muster. They may want to take a breather, while deciding their next step.

If your child wants to pursue college, there are different ways to do that. Some paths may be a better fit for students who are currently undergoing medical treatment. If college isn't the right choice for your child at this point, stay open to other possibilities. You and she may want to explore such alternatives as learning a trade, enrolling in a technical certification program, or getting a job. Whatever direction is chosen, your child still needs support and guidance during the transition to independent adulthood.

What About College?

In my advocacy work, I often hear from parents whose children with Lyme are now heading off to college. In many cases, the child was sick through most of high school and, though much improved, may still be undergoing treatment. Now, he's raring to leave home and start what seems like "real life." Though eager to see their children succeed, these parents may also worry. Will she be able to make it in college, especially if far away from family and support systems? Will he keep up with his medications? What if there is a serious relapse of Lyme symptoms?

These are appropriate and reasonable concerns. They are not the stranglehold of an overprotective parent, although people who don't understand the intricacies of the illness may think so. College life is hectic. New living arrangements, demanding coursework, and a rigorous medical protocol can take a heavy toll. Social pressures to eat junk food, stay up late, drink alcohol, or experiment with drugs don't help. This perfect storm of stress and strain can be overwhelming, and may even result in a serious relapse of Lyme symptoms. Sometimes, students may be forced to drop out of school, and return home ill, discouraged, and aghast at being back in their childhood sick bed.

There are no guarantees that you can prevent this, but there are ways to maximize your child's chances of success. It starts by being realistic about the student's health status. A few questions to consider:

- *Does your student have a complicated regimen of medication, with pills throughout the day and/or IV infusions?* If so, is he up to managing it all himself? If not, what is your back-up strategy? One mom I know counted out her son's medications into a big pill organizer every week and sent it via FedEx to his college dorm. That wouldn't be my choice of how to handle it, but it worked for them. IVs are more complicated. They typically require weekly nursing care to clean the catheter and change the dressing. Are such services available through the college's student health center, or will you have to make other arrangements? Campus clinics may refuse to give any care related to IV medications for chronic Lyme disease, citing the IDSA guidelines.

- *Does the student need ancillary treatments, such as acupuncture or physical therapy?* If so, are you prepared to track down practitioners in the vicinity of the school?

- *How well is your student sleeping?* Sleep is critically important to Lyme patients. College dormitories can be noisy and disruptive. Are single rooms available to freshmen with health problems? Are there other housing options?

Depending on your answers to these questions, you may decide that a school close to home is a better choice than one that's far away. The young person can live on campus, without relinquishing the support of family nearby. Other students may continue to live at home and attend college as a commuter.

In my family's case, Rachel lived at home and attended community college for her first two years. She then transferred to a four-year college out of state. As a freshman, she'd been out of the wheelchair for two years. However, it was still difficult for her to walk long distances or remain standing for any length of time. She was also still taking a lot of medications and other treatments. Beginning college on her own turf, with her home support system in place, minimized the variables. She didn't have to adjust to living on her own, her treatment team was within driving distance, and she still had friends in town.

It also bought us time to figure out a game plan for the future. When she was younger and sicker, I managed her life. I prepared meals, counted pills, made doctor's appointments, and kept track of everything medically related. I cajoled her through her schoolwork, washed her clothes, and maintained the household. Now, her goal was to transfer to a four-year college out-of-state and eventually pursue a career. To carry out such ambitious plans, she would need to take responsibility for her own life. The community college years became a dress rehearsal for living on her own. As had become our style, she ramped up slowly, taking on new tasks one by one. By the time she left for Oregon's Portland State University, she had come a long way. She handled medications, scheduled appointments, and took care of her own medical and personal needs.

Proximity to home isn't the only consideration when selecting a school. For some students, one that's far away can be a good choice if it suits their needs. It's important to be clear-eyed about this when evaluating colleges. For instance, a campus with a lot of steep hills probably isn't a good choice for someone who has difficulty walking. There are many reasons why one college could be better than another for a student with Lyme disease. How close are needed medical services? What are the housing and dining options? What accommodations are available through the college disabilities office?

Disability Services

Many students with Lyme disease shy away from labeling themselves as "disabled." However, the campus disability office is the gateway to many important services. I recommend that students with Lyme register with the disability center even if they don't plan to use it. Then, if the need arises, they are positioned to obtain the supports they require.

Here are academic accommodations that a college might offer:

- Assistive technology, such as tape recorders and screen readers;
- Exam modifications, including extended time on tests and testing in a room with limited distractions;
- Textbooks in alternative formats. Audio books, digital talking books, e-texts, and Braille;
- Note takers, for students whose disabilities make it hard for them to take notes during class.

In grades K-12, schools that receive public funding must identify and provide for the needs of disabled students. Colleges have no such rule. It is up to students to inform the school about their disabilities, if they choose. They must also supply documentation, request accommodations, and advocate for their own needs.

Colleges vary widely in the range of services they offer to disabled students. The University of Illinois, Urbana, provides lift-equipped shuttle bus service both on- and off-campus. San Diego State University makes electric scooters available for short-term loan. The University of Arizona, Tucson, has an adaptive fitness center. It offers exercise equipment designed for people with physical disabilities. You and your student need to identify which services are most important, and look for colleges that offer them.

A young woman I know found out she had Lyme disease shortly before leaving for college. In the middle of her freshman year, she developed eye-related problems that made it difficult for her to read. Through the disability office, she obtained a screen reader for her computer. Here's how she describes it:

> The one I use is called **ReadOutLoud**. It's exactly what it sounds like. It takes web pages, word documents, and text PDFs and reads them out loud to me through my computer. I can adjust the speed of the voice to match how fast I can absorb the words and choose what type of voice it uses. It also has a highlighting/note-taking feature so that I can remember important passages of what I'm reading.

This student uses a wheelchair. She says the school's disability services office has been a lifesaver.

> I literally could not be a college student without them. They give me rides to my classes, help my professors be flexible with my attendance, and give me guides and resources on how to be successful.... Connecting with the disability services office hasn't decreased my independence in any way. In fact, it has provided me with more freedom. Now, I don't have to struggle so much completing basic homework tasks and I can focus more on being successful.

Living Situations

Where will your young adult live while at college? It's a choice that could have huge ramifications for your student's long-term health. When I attended college many years ago, I lived in a dorm room built for two people, with bathrooms down the hall. Because of increased demand for student housing, those same dorms now jam three people into each room. A chronically ill student might find it quite difficult to cope with sharing a room with two others in such cramped quarters. He may be better off in a single room, where he can control the light switch, the sound volume, and the flow of guests in the room.

If you want your child to succeed in college, you need to locate the best living arrangements you can manage. Most colleges offer a range of housing options. I urge you to think carefully about how to optimize your child's chances. Fortunately, my daughter found a single room, with bathroom and kitchenette, in a campus residence hall. She had plenty of social opportunities, but she could also turn off the lights and go to sleep when she needed to. If an emergency arose, there were floor advisors on hand to help.

Not all college students with Lyme are so lucky. Some have been stuck in loud and raucous group living situations that weren't conducive to good eating, sleeping, or studying. (These students were often too embarrassed to let on that they were ill. Maybe the roommates didn't even know there was a problem.) Others with Lyme have gone to the opposite end of the spectrum. They found themselves isolated and alone, too far away from communal buildings to take part in student activities. Look for a middle ground. These students need enough space and autonomy to attend to their personal health, while also being in a position to make friends and take part in campus life. Finding the right balance is essential to a successful college experience.

Dining options also vary by location. Some accommodate different dietary needs and others don't. One student I know bemoaned that the only gluten-free option in her dining hall was iceberg lettuce. If on-campus meals don't work for your student, what are your choices? Standard dorms may allow small refrigerators and microwave ovens. Will that be adequate to your child's needs? If not, are there other possibilities? Some colleges offer on-campus apartments with kitchens. I know someone at an elite private college. She lives in an on-campus house with its own cook, who will make meals for special dietary needs on request.

Tuition Refund Insurance

What if your child's health takes a nosedive in the middle of the school year, and the student is forced to withdraw? Colleges don't typically give refunds for tuition and living expenses. Therefore, you might want to look into whether your child's college offers tuition refund insurance. Make sure you read the fine print, though, since some policies exclude pre-existing medical conditions.

Online Learning

According to a 2013 study, more than 85 percent of colleges and universities in the United States offer at least some classes online. Some offer entire degree programs online, even graduate school programs. Although online learning is an option for chronically ill students, it can be an imperfect solution. "Studying online solves some problems but may create new ones," warns the website of State University of New York's (SUNY) Empire State College. Some students may still need accommodations to get the most out of online courses. According to the SUNY website, areas of difficulty might include:

- comprehending written instructions;
- participating in online discussions;
- viewing and/or hearing online video postings;
- hearing online audio postings; and
- completing assignments on time.

Possible accommodations include extended time for assignments and increased access to the instructor via follow-up emails.

According to *US News and World Report*, some online degree programs are scams. It says the following indicators can help students distinguish a good online program from a bad one:

- Is it accredited?
- Can credits be transferred to another college?
- What support services does the school offer?
- What are its graduation rates?

Like everything else connected with Lyme disease, you and your child must find out what works best for your family. This often means that both the student and the parents must relinquish prior expectations. Perhaps the parents have always wanted their child to go to the same prestigious university they attended. Or maybe the young person has long dreamed about living in a dorm, joining a sorority, or attending school on the other side of the country. It's important to balance such idealized notions with a dose of reality. Assess the challenges and obstacles facing your chronically ill child, and help set him up for success, not failure. Letting go of preconceived ideas may allow you and your child to make the best choices for your situation.

Sandy:

What about those young people for whom college is not a good choice? Here's where the parents and child together need to open their minds to other possibilities.

An example:

Brad was 14 and attending boarding school when he became ill. He returned home, was diagnosed with Lyme disease, and began treatment. For three years he was too sick to go to school. Eventually, he finished high school.

I began working with Brad about the time he enrolled at his local community college. Knowing how much his parents wanted him to continue his schooling, he honored their wishes. But cognitive problems made it hard for him to concentrate and he found the subject matter boring. He tried changing academic directions—first business and then political science. Yet nothing about his classes excited his passion. He passed a few courses and failed others.

Though Brad was intelligent, there were clear gaps in his ability to do his schoolwork. A neuropsychological evaluation was not an option, so he had to figure out his next step without understanding his specific cognitive strengths and weaknesses. Brad became discouraged and decided to give up on college altogether. But what should he do instead? Because he had been ill for most of his teenage years, Brad had no experience to offer future employers and felt insecure about applying for jobs. He went to a couple of interviews and didn't get called back. In my opinion, his lack of confidence was a bigger problem than his lack of job experience.

Then a new coffee shop opened in his area, seeking to hire several employees. Brad interviewed for the job, and to his surprise, he was selected. Working at the coffee shop opened up a whole new world for him. He learned how to satisfy customers and interact well with everyone he encountered throughout the day. He demonstrated an excellent work ethic, always showing up on time and eager to do what needed to be done and he got along well with co-workers. After six months, the boss promoted Brad to shift manager. In that time, he had gone from being an insecure young man who didn't know what he wanted in life to a self-confident supervisor taking satisfaction in a job well done. After about a year at this job, Brad was hired to manage another coffee shop in a large city a few hours away. Moving out of his parents' suburban home opened up social opportunities with people his own age. He successfully bridged the gap from being a sick adolescent to living as an independent adult. He developed the social skills that years of illness had denied him. Perhaps in the future he will return to college. For the moment, however, he's proud of his achievements in the work world and the path he has chosen.

Some young people have no interest in pursuing a four-year academic degree. They should not be pushed into going for an education that would neither satisfy their passions nor provide the kind of learning they enjoy. Other choices exist. Many community colleges offer two-year certificate programs, which prepare students for jobs in areas as diverse as website development, computer networking, cosmetology, graphic design, and photography. There are trade schools that teach auto mechanics and how to repair electrical equipment. Or, some young people might want to find an entry-level job near home and see where things go from there.

Whether chronically ill students plan to attend a four-year college or pursue an alternative, my advice to them is the same. Be clear-eyed about your health needs. Don't bite off more than you can chew. Figure out what it will take to keep you functional and happy, as you work toward goals that are important to you. And whether their young adults are headed to college or taking a different route, my advice to their parents is the same. Support the efforts of your sons and daughters as they embark on this next step towards maturity. Help them make the most of opportunities, while navigating the uncertainties presented by their illness. Show them that you believe in them and want to see their dreams come true.

eleven

Stepping Into The Future

Dorothy:

BY JUNE OF 2008, Rachel was 16 years old and had been in a wheelchair for more than three years. For two of those years, she'd been under the care of a Lyme specialist. After long-term antibiotics and various alternative therapies, many of her symptoms had improved. She could read, think more clearly, and do grade-level schoolwork. No longer consumed by fatigue, she had completed tenth grade, taught herself to produce videos, and was now learning American Sign Language.

However, despite such progress, Rachel still experienced intense, continuous body-wide pain that limited her movement and kept her in the wheelchair. Her shoulders and upper back remained hypersensitive to even the lightest touch. She still could neither sit up straight nor lie down flat. While she could sometimes distract herself from the pain, she could never escape it. Though skilled at hiding her distress, she couldn't keep up that act all the time. Frequently, after an outing, she'd collapse in pain, frustration, and tears. I often felt like collapsing in tears myself.

Then, through a series of coincidences, Rachel talked by phone to a teenage girl she'd never met in person. This girl, whom I will call Michelle, was also in a wheelchair due to Lyme disease. She told Rachel about starting treatment with a specialized chiropractor near San Francisco. After her first session with him, Michelle said, she got up out of her chair and walked a few steps—something she couldn't do before. Rachel begged me to call this new doctor.

I did, and the following week we went to see him. Dr. Andrews[3] performed a thorough examination that included several imaging techniques. This showed that Rachel's neck vertebrae were severely out of alignment, which Dr. Andrews said could affect the central nervous system. He theorized that the Lyme infection may have aggravated an old injury, triggering Rachel's misery. He said it was as if the body had a pain switch that was stuck in the "on" position. Correcting the misalignment could reboot the nervous system like you reboot a computer. With the switch no longer stuck in the on position, her pain might resolve.

None of us knew quite what to make of Dr. Andrews's approach to treatment. It seemed so different from everything else we'd explored in the past three years. But Rachel, my husband, and I were willing to give it a try. Here's how it played out: The first day we saw Dr. Andrews was June 16. Then, three times a week, I drove Rachel two hours to his office. She had an upper cervical chiropractic adjustment, with infrared imaging to monitor progress. Then we drove two hours back home.

We did not see the immediate results that Michelle had reported after her first treatment. Yet, in a few weeks, things began to shift. Rachel's neck didn't hurt as much. In a swimming pool, she could move her arms and legs more freely. By August 1, she could sit

---

3 Not real name

up straight without hurting. A week later, the rest of her pain just seemed to melt away, as Dr. Andrews had predicted. On August 8, Rachel got up out of the wheelchair and walked for the first time in three years.

This happened on a Friday evening, after dinner. We were getting ready to watch the opening ceremonies of the 2008 Beijing Summer Olympics on TV. The Chinese had chosen that date, 08-08-08, because the numbers signified good luck. (08-08-08 certainly brought us good luck!) As it turned out, we missed the televised ceremonies. We held our own Olympic event—walking—at home.

Rachel's limbs were scrawny and out of condition. During her first few tries, they flopped out from under her. But using a walker, then crutches, and then holding onto the crook of my arm, she walked back and forth across our living room. Each step was stronger. Friends came over to witness our miracle, amid tears, and laughter.

The events of 08-08-08 brought us relief and happiness, as well a new, post-wheelchair chapter of our lives. Yet, it's important to point out that this treatment didn't cure Rachel of Lyme disease and co-infections. She continued to have other symptoms that required treatment. But, it removed one huge symptom—constant, incapacitating pain. This made it easier for us to focus on remaining issues. At that time, Dr. Horowitz hadn't yet published *Why Can't I Get Better?* which we mention often in this book. However, his theme pertains directly to Rachel's situation. People with Lyme disease may have many different conditions causing symptoms, and it can take a "medical detective" to ferret them out. Although antibiotics helped Rachel in many ways, I don't think medications alone would have ever alleviated her pain. Misaligned cervical vertebrae were holding her hostage, and we needed a way to release her from their grasp.

About a year after Rachel started walking again, I read a book called *Insights into Lyme Disease Treatment: 13 Lyme-literate Health Care Practitioners Share Their Healing Strategies*, by Connie Strasheim. In one chapter, chiropractor Elizabeth Hesse-Sheehan says, "When the body's structure is misaligned, the nervous system can't deliver the proper signals to the organs and tissues." For some people, she says, fixing structural problems is an essential part of their recovery. In all of my Lyme-related research up to that point, I had never seen that thought expressed. However, since then, I have met many people who report significant relief through such modalities as chiropractic treatment, osteopathic manipulation, physical therapy, craniosacral work, or a manual technique called Lowen Systems. I encourage parents of suffering children to be open to different possibilities. As I learned in my search for answers for Rachel, you have to cast a wide net to find what works for you.

I wish I had definitive answers for the parents who are reading this book. I wish I could tell you that if you followed our instructions, everything would turn out all right. Unfortunately, no such magic recipe exists. But I urge you to keep learning about how this complex illness is affecting your child. Talk to other people in similar circumstances, and use the extensive list of information resources in the back of this book.

Parents of children with Lyme often ask me: Will my child get better? Will she be able to go back to school? Will he ever be able to hold a job? Will our family ever make it out of this deep, dark hole again?

Here's my short answer: Probably. Here's my longer answer: Your child has a good chance of getting substantially better if you

- find a treating doctor who is knowledgeable about Lyme disease and co-infections;

- learn as much as you can about the whole area of Lyme disease and related conditions, so that you can be your child's best advocate;
- learn how to support the immune system with diet and supplements; and
- explore alternative medical options that fit your situation.

In the meantime, do what you can to strengthen your family's emotional and spiritual underpinnings. Don't just focus on the light at the end of the tunnel, which is getting your child well again. Instead, develop ways to bring some light into that tunnel as you all move through it. Find ways to experience happiness and satisfaction, even while coping with difficult circumstances. Find meaning in your life right where you are.

That can be a tall order. Parents of chronically ill children may feel too overwhelmed even to contemplate it. Yet, it's critically important. A book I find helpful is *How to Be Sick: A Buddhist-inspired Guide for the Chronically Ill and Their Caregivers*, by Toni Bernhard. Now, you may be thinking, "Geez. We've already got the 'being sick' part figured out. We don't need any more advice about that." But the book is not about how to get sick or stay sick. It's about how to "be" when you are sick. How to find purpose and joy, even when illness seems to be stealing your life away. Though written from the perspective of a chronically ill adult, its lessons apply to parents of sick children, too. And as you incorporate these helping strategies into your own life, your child will also reap benefits.

Not falling into despair is one of Bernhard's principal themes. She walks readers through her own process for accomplishing that. Some chapter titles include: "Getting Off the Wheel of Suffering," "Facing the Ups and Downs of Chronic Illness with Equanimity," and "The struggle to find community in isolation." (The Internet helps a lot with that last one.) Although I am not a Buddhist, I find Bernhard's insights to be useful and comforting.

Lyme Disease and Groundhog Day

Did you ever see the movie *Groundhog Day*? In this comedy, the character played by actor Bill Murray is caught in a time loop. No matter what he does, he is forced to re-live the same unpleasant day over, and over, and over. Every morning when his clock radio goes off, it is 6 a.m. on February 2, and things unfold exactly the way they did the day before. Nothing he tries can change that. In the hardest stages of my daughter's illness, *Groundhog Day* seemed like an apt metaphor for our lives. We also felt trapped in a time warp, with the same awful script playing out each day. It seemed like we couldn't change anything either. However, unlike Bill Murray's story, our version of Groundhog Day didn't seem funny at all.

Taking each day's "awful script" in stride is one of the challenges of parenting a chronically ill child. You have to strike a balance between facing reality and not becoming so pulled down by it that you can't function. And while you need to have a plan, you can't be thinking too far ahead. For instance, let's say your young teenager is too ill to attend high school. It helps no one if you spend your time obsessing about whether he'll be well enough to attend college in a few years. Better to focus on the present moment. What will it take for you to get through *this* day? What is the next baby step towards wellness? Is there something you and your child can do today that will make you both smile? Is there something you can do for yourself to rest, relax, or relieve stress?

As we hold on to hope that our children will fully recover, it can be heartening to see media coverage of people who have bounced back from Lyme and gone on to great things. One such story is that of freestyle ski champion Angeli VanLaanen. She apparently contracted Lyme disease at age 10, though it wasn't diagnosed at the time. Bouts of illness in her teenage years didn't prevent her from becoming a professional skier. Then, in her 20s, her health collapsed and she had to leave skiing. Finally diagnosed with Lyme disease, she started treatment. After a long and involved process, VanLaanen beat back the illness and returned to her sport.

Her inspiring story is featured in the documentary *Lymelight*. She says she made the film to show others with Lyme that it's possible to get well. After making the movie, VanLaanen won a spot on the US Olympic team, and competed at the 2014 games in Sochi, Russia. Like countless others who followed her thrilling progress, I rolled out of bed early one morning to watch live coverage of the final round. Alas, VanLaanen did not win a medal, placing eleventh overall. But in the eyes of the Lyme community, she had already earned pure gold.

Yet, however much you cheer such success stories, it's important to recognize that your family's circumstances may vary. As your child's health improves, he may play sports again or she may take part in other activities that were once out of reach. Your young adult may be able to finish high school, perhaps go on to college, get a job, and live independently. But is that "cured"? That's hard to say. Relapses can happen. It's essential to remain vigilant even after your child seems well.

Author Jennifer Crystal contracted Lyme disease in her 20s. After years of treatment and a few relapses, she regained her health. As she states in her blog *Jennifer Crystal's Chronicles*,

> *I did not wake up one day and say, "et voilà, I'm all better!" My recovery was more of a spiraling process, with longer stints of good days and then setbacks, and then shorter stints and more setbacks, until the longer reprieves started beating out the shorter ones and the setbacks*

> *became fewer and farther between. This happened over the course of several years, with one major relapse in the middle. But it did happen, and that's not something I could have foreseen, or even believed, when I was in the throes of illness*

> *... I do still have bad days, and when they hit I panic about relapse. But I'm much more resilient now. I rebound much faster... Recovery for people with chronic illness is not about getting back to a pre-illness state; it's about moving forward to a place where Lyme and other diseases are part of a functioning life.*

Most of the people I know who have gotten their lives back after chronic Lyme—both adults and children—tend to be more like Crystal and less like VanLaanen. Their situation improves in fits and starts, with detours along the way. Even those who no longer require medication must still be mindful about their health. They can't ignore sleep, nutrition, and exercise. They must avoid exposure to mold and other environmental toxins. They may never reach a point at which they can be blissfully oblivious to such concerns. Day-to-day life may never again look exactly like it did before they got sick. But it can be a good life nonetheless.

Lyme Disease Advocacy as a Healing Strategy

As my family went through its hardest days with my daughter, I coped by spending as much time as possible online, looking for answers. As I learned more about this complex topic, it became glaringly obvious that Lyme was so much more than a scientific and medical puzzle. It was also a political quagmire. Strong factions had vested interests in keeping the status quo, while multitudes of people with Lyme disease were abandoned by officials who are supposed to guard the public health. Furthermore, news coverage of Lyme-related issues was meager. (This was 2005-2007. It has increased significantly since then.) As I pondered this frustrating situation, I felt defeated, helpless, and angry. I could not envision what it would take to change the dynamic. Partly this was because the convoluted issues were so hard to explain to people who weren't living the experience themselves.

Then, one day, I saw an item online about San Francisco filmmaker Andy Abrahams Wilson, who was shooting a documentary about Lyme disease called *Under Our Skin*. The write-up captured my imagination immediately. I could see the possibilities. A well-made film could garner national media attention and help bring the message to a large audience.

Enthralled by the idea, I emailed Wilson, asking if there was anything I could do from a distance to help. I told him that although I was confined to the house tending a very sick child, I was "pretty good at using Google." To my surprise, Wilson sent me a research project—sifting through online archives for Lyme-related news coverage. I worked on it at night while my daughter slept. Mine was a small contribution, but it gave me satisfaction to play even a minor part in what turned out to be an amazing, award-winning film. Furthermore, those late night Internet research sessions marked my entry into the world of Lyme disease advocacy. I was no longer only trying to help my own family. Being connected to a larger cause broke the vicious cycle of my personal Groundhog Day.

Under Our Skin was a game-changer for the Lyme community. It powerfully illustrated the plight of people with Lyme disease and the controversy surrounding it. Moreover, the film became a rallying point for Lyme patients and a gateway to activism. Hundreds of community showings of *Under Our Skin* sprang up throughout the United States and Canada (and eventually around the world.) Frequently, these screenings brought news coverage, often featuring local people with

Lyme disease and depicting their difficulties in finding treatment. This brought home the message that Lyme disease was something happening to "regular folks" in neighborhoods across the continent. Eventually, *Under Our Skin* was shown on national television in the United States, and is now available for free viewing online. In 2014, Wilson brought out a sequel, *Under Our Skin 2: Emergence.*

The release of *Under Our Skin* coincided with a social development that had huge implications for Lyme disease advocacy—the rise of Facebook. Suddenly, here was an easy way for Lyme patients and their advocates to connect with each other, while sharing news and information about Lyme disease. Facebook pages for *Under Our Skin*, LymeDisease.org, the Lyme Disease Association (LDA) and other advocacy groups became important channels of communication. They became a place for individuals to find out they were not alone, and that by joining with others they might bring about change.

Facebook wasn't the beginning of Lyme disease advocacy, of course. That had started years earlier when individuals in different places started speaking up about Lyme disease. One of them was Phyllis Mervine, from rural Northern California. Mervine became chronically ill in 1977, and suffered a range of bizarre symptoms for ten years before being diagnosed with Lyme. After several years of treatment, she was able to function again.

In those pre-Internet days, she remembers, there was no place for patients to learn anything about this newly recognized disease. So, in 1989, Mervine started a publication called *The Lyme Times*. Its first issue was two legal-sized sheets of paper folded into a booklet. As it grew, it included articles by doctors, researchers and laypeople, as well as contact information for support groups. "Besides educating people, we wanted to bring them together and empower them," Mervine recalls. She hoped that reading stories about Lyme patient activism might inspire others to get involved despite their own illness. Today, *The Lyme Times* is a well-respected journal that is mailed all over the world and available online to members of LymeDisease.org.

Another early advocate who is still going strong is Patricia Smith of the Lyme Disease Association (LDA). In the 1980s, when she was a school board member in Wall Township, New Jersey, local students and teachers were contracting a little known disease called Lyme.

> *I wanted to learn everything I could about the disease to prevent my children and others from getting it. I did not understand how my district could have dozens of sick kids and staff and no one knew anything or told the district anything. All these people were going into the local hospital getting IVs, having seizures, yet it was almost as though it were top secret, nobody was distributing any information about the disease, not the health department, not the hospital.*

Smith kept digging, and eventually obtained information from the US Navy, which had documented early cases of Lyme at a base in New Jersey. She distributed this material throughout the school district. In time, her advocacy broadened from her local area to the whole state of New Jersey.

Within a few years, two of Smith's daughters started showing symptoms of the disease, and it was a fight to get them diagnosed and treated.

> *All the while I did local advocacy. In the mid-90s when I did my first ever picket at a NJ hospital where the doctor there was preventing treatment for Lyme, and my daughter was in 18-hour-long temporal lobe seizures six to seven days a week, for a three year period, I came home to find her in the fetal position and totally non-communicative. I made a vow that day that if she recovered, I would never let another mother go through what I had been through alone. I have tried to keep that vow.*

205

Smith's New Jersey organization eventually went national, with chapters and affiliates in many states. In her role as LDA president, Smith has raised money for research, educated local, state and federal policymakers, testified for legislation, organized conferences with international speakers, written educational materials, published professional journal articles, and has spoken at hundreds of public, school, business, and government events.

Where Does This Story Continue?

Sandy:

I have never met a single person who, if given the option, would choose to have Lyme disease or to see their child have it. I have never met anyone who didn't wish they had been diagnosed early, when it would have been easier to treat. But we weren't given that choice. So we look at this Lyme journey we take and wonder where the road will lead us.

We have been compelled to travel a path that is not well understood. The illness isolates us. Choosing treatment that's out of the medical mainstream may isolate us, and our families, even more. Parents worry about whether their children will ever recover and what their lives will be like in the future. While we know a lot more about treatment options for chronic tick-borne diseases than we did when I was first diagnosed in 1990, there are no guarantees. We don't know how long treatment will take and what it will cost in lost months or years of childhood.

Similar to survivors of other traumas, children and families may find that the world is a different place after their experience of chronic Lyme disease. Even those who fully recover find that they may not go back to the life they once knew, because they aren't the same people they were before. Interestingly, many feel that this change is for the better.

One ninth-grade girl was out of school for about two years, too ill to keep up with friends. She found movie theaters too loud, and even just hanging out at someone's house was too tiring. When she recovered enough to return to school, she was eager to connect with her old classmates. Yet, when she finally saw them, she was sorely disappointed. Her world view had shifted, and she had no patience for all the gossip and drama over what she saw as little things. She wasn't glad that she had had Lyme, but going through the experience helped her embrace a new, more mature way of looking at life. She now sought out people who cared more about others and about making a difference in the world. I told her that in my view, her personal growth and new values were among what I consider the "gifts of Lyme." She agreed.

One young man had turned to homeschooling after the school district refused to meet his needs. Those years when he was severely disabled allowed him the time and opportunity to make movies on his computer. He's now doing very well in a highly respected film program at a major university. Another gift of Lyme.

Many families that I've seen would never have sought therapy had their child not been ill. Yet, when Lyme forced their hand, they realized that their family needed to learn to communicate more effectively, so they could pull together and function as a team. Working through these issues in therapy helped them understand the meaning of sacrifice and shared values, while strengthening the family bonds.

This book has been about dealing with kids that are ill. But what happens when your child starts getting well? That's the outcome you've been dreaming of, right? The symptoms resolve, your son or daughter resumes school and other activities, and life returns to normal. Or does it?

Those of us who have struggled with Lyme ourselves or with our family members know that there is no definite way to tell that it is really over. After Lyme has invaded our families, we can never again feel carefree about it. It's an uncertainty that we live with, day after day, after day.

So, even if things seem good with your child, maybe one day a troublesome symptom pops up. Her knee hurts, she has difficulty concentrating, or she seems extra tired. This terrifies you. Is Lyme rearing its ugly head again? It's natural for parents who have lived through such a traumatic experience to hit the panic button if something looks remotely Lyme-related. But I encourage you not to immediately assume the worst. Stay calm and pay close attention to what's going on. Then, if the situation requires it, you'll be better prepared to take action.

We want our kids to live their young lives to the fullest and to enjoy the new adventures, challenges, and friendships of youth. We don't want them to be constantly in fear of the future. We can help them accomplish this by modeling the same qualities ourselves. I suggest that you take to heart the slogan "one day at a time." Live in the present, being grateful for the gifts of the day—your child's return to health, and all the activities that allows. Drink in the enjoyment of this new phase of your life.

This doesn't mean you won't pay heed to signs of a possible relapse, because you know about Lyme and the issues it brings. Your hard-won experience will stand you in good stead. You will never again be in the position you were in when Lyme symptoms first hit, when you had no idea what was wrong with your child. You know where to find the right treatment and support, as well as how to engage with the medical community.

Thus, I urge you to greet every morning as a new day. Do what needs to be done, and learn what needs to be learned. Don't burden yourself with worry about what is still to come. You and your family can get past the trials and tribulations of this moment, fostering a resilience that will carry you though to the future. My hope is that you will not only survive Lyme disease, but triumph over it.

Afterword

Dorothy and Sandy:

It is a bitter reality that many of this book's recommendations are financially out of reach to some of the very people who need them the most. This is a consequence of the harsh political climate surrounding Lyme disease in the medical world. As we have discussed in preceding chapters, the current system makes it challenging to get diagnosed and even harder to find helpful treatment. Furthermore, many families find it difficult to obtain insurance coverage for extended Lyme treatment. Thus, to get the care they need, patients must often pay out of pocket—and those pockets can wear thin in a very short time. There are a few sources of financial assistance for people with Lyme disease, which we list in Appendix A. Alas, how we wish the list were longer.

At this stage, there are no easy fixes for the toll that Lyme disease takes on individuals and society at large. Here are some things that need to happen in order for things to start moving in the right direction:

- **Better education** so people can learn how to prevent Lyme and other tick-borne diseases in the first place.
- **Better diagnostic tools for identifying early Lyme,** when it's easiest to treat.
- **Better diagnostic tools for identifying chronic tick-borne illnesses,** starting with official recognition of this complex set of conditions.
- **Releasing doctors from the stranglehold of the IDSA Lyme guidelines,** which trivialize the suffering of people who don't fit into its neat categories and stand in the way of appropriate diagnosis and treatment.
- **Better medical treatments for Lyme** in both its acute and chronic forms.
- **Better reporting**, so that local, state and federal health officials can gain an accurate picture of the true extent of Lyme and other tick-borne diseases, in order to adequately respond to them.
- **Insurance coverage for long-term treatment of Lyme and other tick-borne illnesses.** Individuals should not have to bankrupt their families in order to get the care they need.

This will require a major transformation in how our government views and handles the serious threat posed by Lyme disease. Fueled by the energy of individuals who have been touched by Lyme disease, patient advocacy organizations are laboring to help change this situation. Many of them are listed in the following resource section. We urge our readers to learn more about the work of these groups and to contribute to their efforts in any way that they can. If Lyme patients and their families link arms together, we can help build a world in which children—and everybody else—are freed from the scourge of Lyme disease. Won't you join us in this important work?

Appendices

Appendix A—Resource List

Lyme Education, Advocacy, Support, and Fundraising Organizations

Bay Area Lyme Foundation raises money to fund research into better diagnosis and treatment for Lyme disease. www.bayarealyme.org

Children's Lyme Disease Network is dedicated to raising awareness of how Lyme and other tick-borne illnesses affect children, specifically. Website includes information about PANS/PANDAS. www.childrenslymenetwork.org

Family Connections Center for Counseling is the website of family therapist Sandra Berenbaum, LCSW, BCD, co-author of this book. It includes information for families dealing with Lyme disease, as well as first-person accounts of children with Lyme disease. www.lymefamilies.com

Global Lyme Alliance (GLA) was recently formed by the merger of the Tick-Borne Diseases Association and Lyme Research Alliance. GLA raises money for Lyme disease research and has an informative website. www.globallymealliance.com

International Lyme and Associated Diseases Society (ILADS) is a professional organization for physicians and other healthcare providers who treat Lyme disease. It sponsors medical and scientific conferences in the United States and abroad. The ILADS website is a useful source of Lyme-related information, including downloadable brochures. www.ilads.org

Lyme Connection—This Connecticut organization sponsors educational events for the general public, as well as specialized sessions for mental health practitioners. The group has developed an innovative Lyme disease prevention program called BLAST, which has received state funding. Informative website and YouTube channel. www.lymeconnection.org

LymeDisease.org, a national advocacy organization, is a leading source for news, information, and analysis in the Lyme community. Its website has information about ticks, Lyme disease, co-infections, prevention, risk maps, and more. The quarterly print journal, *The Lyme Times*, is sent free to members. It also offers a network of online support groups, free email newsletters, Facebook and Twitter updates, as well as the *Lyme Policy Wonk* and *Touched by Lyme* blogs. www.lymedisease.org

Lyme Disease Association raises funds for research, works to promote Lyme-related legislation on both the federal and state levels, has chapters and affiliates in many states, cosponsors patient education workshops, and puts on an annual scientific conference in conjunction with Columbia University. The website has a doctor referral tool. www.lymediseaseassosciation.org

Mental Health and Illness—This website contains the writings of psychiatrist Robert Bransfield, MD, a foremost expert on how Lyme disease affects the brain. www.mentalhealthandilllness.com

National Capitol Lyme Disease Association—Education and support activities, primarily focused in the greater Washington, DC, area. www.natcaplyme.org

The Human Side of Lyme—The research and writings of Dr. Virginia Sherr, a Pennsylvania psychiatrist with a special interest in the neurocognitive symptoms of Lyme disease. www.thehumansideoflyme.net

Financial Grants for Children With Lyme Disease

LymeAid4Kids—For those under age 21 without insurance coverage for Lyme disease, this program provides up to $1,000 towards diagnosis and treatment. It was created by author Amy Tan in conjunction with the Lyme Disease Association. See www.lymediseaseassociation.org for an application package.

Lymelight Foundation—Financial grants for Lyme treatment for patients from birth to age 25, up to a lifetime maximum of $10,000. Grants cover expenses relating to the treatment of Lyme disease, including medication, supplements, doctor visits, lab testing, alternative practitioners, such as acupuncturists and chiropractors, and transportation to and from an out-of-area doctor or lab. www.lymelightfoundation.org

Lyme-TAP—Lyme Test Access Program offers financial assistance for Lyme and tick-borne disease diagnostic testing. It will reimburse up to 75 percent of out-of-pocket costs of testing from a qualified CLIA/Medicare-approved laboratory of your choice. (US residents only; not limited to children) www.lymetap.com

Other Financial Assistance

NeedyMeds—This website offers free information on programs that help people who can't afford medications and healthcare. It also provides information on financial assistance for prescription medicines, low-cost medical and dental clinics, drug discount cards, and information about Medicare and Medicaid. www.needymeds.org

Prescription Hope—You pay a monthly fee for this service, which helps you obtain low-cost medications. www.prescriptionhope.com

Information About PANS/PANDAS

PANDAS Resource Network
www.pandasresourcenetwork.org

PANDAS Network
www.pandasnetwork.org

Latitudes
www.latitudes.org

International OCD Foundation
www.iocdf.org

Online Support Groups

Lymeparents
https://groups.yahoo.com/neo/groups/Lymeparents/info

Lyme and pregnancy Facebook group
https://www.facebook.com/groups/492653780749584/

LymeDisease.org's network of state-based support groups
http://www.lymedisease.org/get-involved/take-action/find-your-state-group/

Lymenet.org online discussion groups

MDJunction has a variety of online health support groups, including Lyme disease and Parents of Children with Lyme. www.MDJunction.com

Facebook has hundreds of Lyme-related pages and groups.

Books About Lyme Disease and Related Topics

The Beginner's Guide to Lyme Disease by Nicola McFadzean, ND. (Biomed Publishing, 2012.) An overview of the illness, the controversy, and treatment options.

Coping with Lyme Disease: A Practical Guide to Dealing with Diagnosis and Treatment by Denise Lang, with Kenneth Liegner, MD. (Holt Paperbacks, 3rd Edition, 2004)

Cure Unknown: Inside the Lyme Epidemic by Pamela Weintraub (St. Martin's Griffin, 2nd Edition, 2013), a medical journalist whose whole family has had Lyme disease, delves into the scientific, medical, and political turmoil surrounding the illness.

Digging Deep: A Journal for Young People Facing Health Challenges by Rose Offner and Sheri Sobrato Brisson. (Resonance House, 2014)

Infusing for Lymies, free online book with lots of information about IV drugs and PICC lines. http://issuu.com/lymeunderground/docs/infusingforlymies

The Lyme Diet by Dr. Nicola McFadzean (Biomed Publishing, 2010). Nutritional strategies for healing from Lyme disease. What to eat while healing from Lyme.

The Lyme Disease Solution by Dr. Kenneth Singleton (Booksurge, 2008). An introduction to the medical aspects of Lyme diagnosis and treatment.

My Lyme Guide by Marjorie MacArthur Veiga and Sarah Fletcher, MD (My Lyme Guide, 2013). This book provides organizational tools for patients and caregivers for tracking symptoms, medications, insurance records, and more. MyLymeGuide.com

Suffering the Silence: Chronic Lyme Disease in an Age of Denial by Allie Cashel (North Atlantic Books, 2015). Written by a young woman who became infected with Lyme when she was 7 years old.

Out of the Woods: Healing from Lyme disease for Body, Mind and Spirit by Katina Makris (Helios Press, 2015). This memoir, written from an adult perspective, includes a lot of information about integrative and alternative methods of healing. Makris also blogs, gives workshops, and hosts Lymelight Radio. www.katinamakris.com

Why Can't I Get Better? Solving the Mystery of Lyme and Chronic Disease by Dr. Richard Horowitz (St. Martin's Press, 2013). One of the most comprehensive books about treating Lyme disease and other factors that may accompany it. See more about the book and download Dr. Horowitz's five-page symptom questionnaire at the website www.CanGetBetter.com.

Videos

Under Our Skin and *Under Our Skin 2: Emergence*—These two documentaries demonstrate the profound effect of Lyme disease on patients and explain the complex politics of tick-borne illness in the United States. The original book can be viewed online for no charge on Hulu and YouTube. The sequel can be viewed online for a small charge. Details at www.underourskin.com

Educating Your Child With Lyme Disease

Council of Parent Attorneys and Advocates (COPAA) is a nonprofit network of attorneys, advocates, parents and related professionals to protect the legal and civil rights of students with disabilities.

CHADD—Children and Adults with Attention-Deficit/Hyperactivity Disorder provides education, advocacy and support for individuals with ADHD. Informative website and a variety of printed materials.

Home School Legal Defense Association is a nonprofit advocacy organization providing homeschooling-related legal advice and resources. Includes a clickable map of the United States, with information about homeschooling laws in each state. www.hslda.org

Homeschool.com offers resources, information, and message boards.

OnlyPassionateCuriosity.com is a homeschooling blog with lots of advice and resource links.

Specialeducationguide.com includes a useful "special education dictionary," explaining terms parents may need to know in dealing with schools.

Wrightslaw offers information about special education law, education law, and advocacy for children with disabilities. Parents can sign up to receive regular e-mails related to education advocacy, location of Wrightslaw seminars, available books. We recommend *From Emotions to Advocacy—The Special Education Survival Guide*, 2nd Edition by Pam Wright and Pete Wright. More information at www.wrightslaw.com.

Other Resources

Direct Access Labs

Most states allow direct access testing (DAT), which allows you to obtain standard lab tests without a doctor's order and pay substantially less than you might otherwise pay. More information at the following websites:

www.accesalabs.com

www.directlabs.com

www.privatemdlabs.com

www.walkinlab.com

www.health-tests-direct.com

Disability-Related Resources

Beach wheelchairs in California:
www.coastal.ca.gov/access/beach-wheelchairs.html

Beach wheelchairs on the East Coast and other places: www.beachwheelchair.com/rentals.htm

United Disability Services offers lots of information about how to modify a home for various disabilities. www.estore.udservices.org

The US government's website on resources and services for those with disabilities includes information about modifying homes for accessibility. www.Disability.gov

Food Allergies

Food Allergy Research and Education (FARE)
www.foodallergy.org

Celiac Disease Foundation offers extensive information about gluten-free diets, including menu plans. www.Celiac.org

Lyme-Related Vision Problems

The Padula Institute of Vision's website provides information about visual processing disorders and other eye problems related to Lyme disease. www.padulainstitute.com.

Media Reviews

Common Sense Media provides independent ratings and reviews for movies, games, apps, TV shows, websites, books, and music. www.commonsensemedia.com

Smartphone Apps

Medications: Pillboxie, Pill Reminder, Drugs.com

Symptom trackers: My Pain Diary, Symple, iMoodJournal, Period Tracker

Other record keeping: Paperless, Keep

Gluten-free Restaurants: Find Me Gluten Free, iEatOut Gluten and Allergen Free

Public Restrooms: The Bathroom Map, Where to Wee

Appendix B

Selections From the *Touched by Lyme* Blog

Dorothy Leland's blog, *Touched by Lyme*, explores the personal side of Lyme disease and how it affects individuals and families. It also highlights useful information for people seeking answers about this complicated illness. To read the whole blog and/or to sign up for email notifications of new blog posts, go to www.lymedisease.org.

TOUCHED BY LYME: How to protect yourself in tick territory

Ticks can be found in different kinds of terrain, at different times of the year, in different kinds of weather. Many are quite small, as easily overlooked as a speck of dirt. They tend to be near the ground—in decomposing leaves, grass, bushes, fallen logs, and on the lower part of tree trunks. When you brush by them, they may transfer to your shoe, your pant leg, or your arm. Sometimes ticks hitch a ride on your dog's fur. And then come on over to you when they get the chance.

A tick may walk up your clothing until it can access skin. When it strikes, it embeds its mouth parts in you and starts sucking your blood. The longer a tick is attached to the body, the more likely it will transmit disease. When engorged with your blood, the tick swells up to the size of a raisin.

Different kinds of ticks can carry different diseases. Your best defense against all tick-borne illness is avoiding tick exposure in the first place. Your second best defense is to quickly find and remove any ticks that latch on to you.

Most people who contract Lyme get it from a nymphal (immature) tick. Because nymphs are as small as poppy seeds and their bite is painless, many people don't notice or remove them.

An excellent way to protect yourself is to wear insect-repellent clothing. The fabric has been treated with a special process that binds permethrin (a repellent) to the fibers. Testing has shown it to be highly effective against ticks, mosquitoes, ants, flies, chiggers, and midges. Protection lasts through at least 70 washings. Alternatively, you can buy an aerosol can of permethrin at outdoor stores and treat your clothing yourself, which will last through five or six washings.

It's important to protect your feet. One study showed that people with permethrin-treated footwear had 74 times the protection of those without it. When you spray your shoes or boots, do it outside in a well-ventilated area, making sure you don't breathe the vapors.

You should also apply insect repellent to exposed skin. Studies show that repellents that include DEET, picaridin, or lemon eucalyptus oil are most effective.

While in the field, check yourself periodically for ticks. Use fine-tipped tweezers to remove any embedded ticks you may find. (Don't douse them with lighter fluid, dish soap, or other such "remedies." That can make the tick regurgitate its contents into you—not what we're going for here.)

When you come in for the day, running your clothing through a hot dryer (before you wash them) for at least 10 minutes will kill any live ticks that might be present in your clothing. Then, take a shower and thoroughly check your entire body. As you run soapy hands over your skin, feel for unexpected bumps, which might be embedded ticks. Pay special attention to hidden spots—behind the ears, hairline, armpits, groin, and belly button. Parents should check their young children.

Whether or not you find a tick, stay alert for symptoms that could arise from a tick-borne illness. A bull's-eye rash indicates Lyme disease, but not everybody with Lyme gets one. You might have a different rash or none at all. You may develop flu-like symptoms—fever, headache, nausea—or joint pain or dizziness.

Ticks can carry all kinds of nasty stuff—not just Lyme disease. For more information about Lyme and other tick-borne infections, go to www.lymedisease.org.   —*July 27, 2015*

TOUCHED BY LYME: *Known tick bite, no symptoms, what to do?*

I recently received the following message: My 3-year-old grandson, who lives in Westchester, NY, had a tick discovered in his scalp last week. We are not sure how long it was there but the last time he was near some trees or shrubs or grass was four days before. My son removed it and sent it to a lab for examination. It was a "partially engorged" adult female deer tick, which tested positive for Lyme. He is presently asymptomatic, but what is the prevalent thinking on treatment at this point?

My reply: "Partially engorged" means that it must have been on your grandson for a while. Plenty of time, unfortunately, to transmit pathogens. I recommend you get in touch with a local Lyme support group for advice on where you could take him in your area. (*Then I listed some.*)

His reply: Thank you for your response. Should an asymptomatic (after less than a week) 3-year-old be treated with antibiotics prophylactically after being found with a positive deer tick on his scalp (probably there for 3 – 4 days)? What is the current treatment protocol?

My reply: I'm not a doctor and this should not be construed as medical advice. I'm writing to you parent-to-parent. Your grandson lives in one of the most highly Lyme-endemic regions in the country. That area also has a high rate of babesia, another serious illness that can be transmitted along with Lyme during a single tick bite. You know the boy was bitten by a tick that was infected with at least one dangerous microbe. It might have carried several more. Some people who are infected with tick-borne diseases show symptoms right away. Others may not show symptoms for months or even years. Yet early treatment is your best chance to knock the bad bugs out of the ballpark. Otherwise, they can burrow deep into the body, cause all kinds of hurt and be extremely difficult to get rid of.

You ask about the current treatment protocol. Well, that depends on who you ask. Some doctors, following the lead of the Infectious Diseases Society of America's Lyme treatment guidelines, might tell you to watch and wait to see if the child develops a bull's-eye rash or other manifestations of Lyme. But by the time symptoms show up, you will have lost that precious window of opportunity to get the upper hand on the spirochetes before they get the upper hand on you. Many children suffer lifelong disability because their parents followed a doctor's advice to watch and wait for symptoms to develop.

All I can tell you is what I would do if I found myself in your place. I'd move heaven and earth to get my little guy to a Lyme-literate MD, affiliated with the International Lyme and Associated Diseases Society (ILADS). They sometimes have a long waiting list for appointments. But many of them, if you say your child has recently been bitten by a tick that tested positive for Lyme, will give you a "recent tick bite appointment" right away. Then, you can explore treatment options with somebody who understands the importance of not passively waiting for symptoms to show up.   —*April 2, 2014*

TOUCHED BY LYME: Lyme, MCS & getting a driver's license

Getting a driver's license is a rite of passage that young people with chronic Lyme disease sometimes miss. If you're too sick to even get out of bed, you can't very well practice parallel parking, can you?

When somebody that ill finally feels better, getting a driver's license is often number one on their to-do list.

But sometimes, even if you're well enough to drive, other issues get in the way.

A young woman I'll call "Sally" has been dealing with Lyme and multiple chemical sensitivities (MCS) for many years. This made her miss out on a number of teen milestones, including getting a driver's license. She's in her 20s now, her health has improved in some ways, and she has learned to drive a car.

But MCS remains a huge barrier. Among other things, she reacts badly to scented products such as shampoo, deodorant, and laundry detergent. She can't be in close quarters with anybody using them. She'll get a horrible migraine, her lungs will start to burn, and she'll feel stabbing liver pains.

"Taking a driving test can be nerve wracking for anybody," Sally told me. "But for someone who reacts to fragrances, taking a test next to someone wearing scented products would be impossible. There's no way I could pass my test under those conditions."

Sally and her mom contacted the California Department of Motor Vehicles with what might have seemed like an odd request. Could they arrange for a test examiner to use special shampoo and soap and deodorant that Sally wouldn't react to? It was the only thing that would work for her.

Unfortunately, the first DMV employee they talked to wasn't helpful. He made it sound like her request required mountains of paperwork, medical documentation, and bureaucratic hoops.

But that wasn't the end of the story. Phone calls made to DMV headquarters in Sacramento landed on more sympathetic ears and things fell into place.

Sally dropped off a bag of fragrance-free products (shampoo, conditioner, deodorant) at her local DMV office. The examiner took them home and used them before the day of the test. Sally's appointment was scheduled for 7:30 a.m., before the office opened, to reduce her exposure to other people. She took the test and passed with flying colors.

It's an example of how a little bit of accommodation by others can make a big difference in the life of somebody with MCS. I applaud the DMV for its flexibility and I doff my hat to the test examiner who was willing to change shampoo and deodorant to help the cause.

Sally says the freedom to drive has brought a breath of fresh air into her life. "I no longer have to depend on my parents for transportation. I have taken another step toward my independence."

And isn't that what we wish for every chronic Lyme patient— the chance to finally get on with their lives? —*April 1, 2012*

Appendix C

Excerpts of Articles by Sandra Berenbaum

From *The Lyme Times*, Summer, 2005:

Reflections on Lyme Disease in the Family

A child's illness may call on parents to grow in unaccustomed ways. Parents may find themselves thrust into situations beyond their own comfort level, needing to be more assertive with previously trusted school and medical authority figures or more conciliatory with insurers and others, in order to achieve important goals. The needs of their children often push parents far beyond their comfort zone in these areas. It is important that parents recognize where that comfort zone is, and work to move beyond it, for the sake of their child, and his recovery.

In this complex, demanding world, we need to have compassion, empathy, and understanding for those who are struggling to raise children who have chronic Lyme disease. If we can appreciate the challenges that face them, and respect their decisions, perhaps we can make their world a little bit brighter.

Parenting Strategies From the Trenches

After years of helping parents, children, adolescents, and families deal with some of these issues, I have developed the following strategies, to help parents ease their journey:

- Maintain a problem-focused approach as you make decisions about diagnosis, doctors, and treatment.
- Work at developing a consensus between you and your child's other parent, whether or not you are still together!

- Stay focused on current problems to be solved, and keep worries on the back burner.

- Explain what's going on to your child in concrete, age-appropriate terms.

- Maintain your credibility with your child by being truthful.

- Be careful with the words you use. Avoid words like "psychotic episode," "manic," or "incurable." Lyme disease is a scary illness. Keep your words from making it scarier.

- Be firm when you need to be, but give choices when you can, lots of choices.

- Establish and maintain protective boundaries, protecting yourself and your child from family members and friends who doubt your judgment and parenting decisions. Let others know what they can and cannot say.

- Build a supportive network—educate your family and friends about Lyme, but don't overload them. Remember, this is your issue, not theirs.

- Be open to support, but make it clear that you're not open to being second-guessed. Allow people to help in concrete ways when you're overwhelmed. Let them make meals, pick up the kids, or shop for groceries.

From *The Lyme Times,* Fall/Winter Issue 2002/3

Kids and Lyme: How it Affects Their Learning

Here are some of the accommodations that might be put into place, and how I've seen children helped by these accommodations. Some may require that a neuropsychological evaluation document the particular learning problem that leads to the need for the accommodation.

- Unlimited time for testing—a child is afforded extended time to take tests. Some children with Lyme have problems with the speed of processing information. These children get exceedingly anxious, trying to take a timed test. This accommodation removes the anxiety, literally gives them enough time to think.

- Separate testing location—this is appropriate for children who have problems with focusing and concentration, and are easily distracted. There are fewer children taking the test, in a quiet location.

- Tests read to student—this is for students who have particular verbal learning problems, in which their auditory learning is less impaired than their visual learning.

- Excused from a percentage of their homework. Children with profound fatigue, who have a difficult time just getting through the school day, benefit greatly from having less work to do at home.

Keep in mind that *more* school work is not necessarily *better*. If a child is fatigued and has problems with memory and organization, of what use is hours of homework, at the end of the school day, or on the weekend? Of what benefit is increasing the child's anxiety by requiring that he/she perform equal to the children who are well? Are they really being treated equally, if the child who is well can do the work in one-quarter to one-half the time as the child who is ill? Shouldn't the sick child have at least an equal right to down time, time to relax, and recover, to face the next learning challenge?

(Complete version of these articles and others by Sandy Berenbaum are available on her website, www.lymefamilies.com.)

Appendix D

Berenbaum Lyme Disease Screening Protocol

During my years of working in this field, I came to recognize that mental health practitioners need a simple screening tool that might help them identify Lyme disease symptoms. They could then refer the patient to a Lyme-knowledgeable medical practitioner for evaluation, diagnosis and treatment. I developed this protocol, which has also proved useful to patients and parents.

—Sandy Berenbaum

1. History of changes in:
   - behavior at home, school, or in other settings
   - school performance or attendance
   - sleeping and eating patterns
   - socialization patterns, or dramatic change in peer group
   - sensory sensitivity (light, sound, taste, texture)
   - mood
     - o depression
     - o anxiety
     - o suicidal ideation or gestures
     - o new onset or intensification of PMS
     - o new onset obsessive compulsive disorder (OCD)
2. History of changes in activity level, that could be suggestive of Lyme disease: Sudden loss of interest, or inability to participate in activities, such as organized sports, music, dance, drama, youth group, etc.;
3. A discrete point in time at which problems began;

4. History of onset of other psychiatric symptoms (panic attacks, OCD, hallucinations, cognitive and executive functioning problems) not present in early childhood;

5. History of use of psychiatric medications, with either no success in symptom reduction or a paradoxical response;

6. History of any physical illness (flu, mononucleosis, bronchitis) occurring prior to start of psychiatric, learning or behavioral problems;

7. History of short-term antibiotic treatment for medical problem (strep infection, etc.) with temporary improvement of other symptoms.

Appendix E—Background About The IDSA Lyme Disease Guidelines

Reprinted by permission of LymeDisease.org

In 2013, the United States Centers for Disease Control and Prevention (CDC) made headlines by releasing new estimates of how many people are infected with Lyme disease every year. They increased the number ten-fold, from 30,000 to 300,000. However, nothing has changed about how Lyme disease is diagnosed and treated. Or, more often, *not* diagnosed and *not* treated.

Untold thousands of Lyme patients across the United States are denied access to appropriate medical care because the CDC promulgates Lyme treatment guidelines put forth by the Infectious Diseases Society of America (IDSA). The IDSA is a private medical association that doesn't have to answer to anybody. The CDC is a federal agency that essentially allows the IDSA to set its policy regarding Lyme disease.

Medical treatment guidelines are tremendously important. Guidelines for most diseases are listed by the National Guidelines Clearinghouse (NGC), which is part of the US Department of Health and Human Services. It's the government's way of providing updated information to health care professionals. Doctors consult guidelines to help them determine how best to treat their patients, and insurance companies use them to decide what treatments to pay for.

The Current IDSA Lyme Guidelines Misrepresent Science and Restrict Access to Care

The IDSA defines the illness so narrowly that many people otherwise determined to have Lyme disease are denied access to medical care. Even those given treatment are usually limited to a "standard course" of antibiotics (often two-to-three weeks), even when they remain ill. Furthermore, insurance companies often won't pay for anything beyond what's stipulated in the guidelines.

Examples of How the IDSA Guidelines Misrepresent or Ignore Science

- They state that only "a few" patients remain ill after standard treatment, while the true figure is 25 to 50 percent. (Stricker & Johnson 2011)
- They say the NIH-funded trials prove definitively that longer treatments are not effective, *despite the fact* that only four such human studies have been conducted, *despite the fact* that two of the studies showed improvement on treatment, and *despite the fact* that the sample populations in each of the treatment trials was small and did not reflect patients seen in clinical practice (Delong et al. 2012, Fallon et al. 2012). Fallon's evaluation of the four trials concludes that "approximately 60 percent of patients with persistent post-treatment Lyme fatigue may experience meaningful but partial clinical improvement in fatigue with antibiotic retreatment."
- Two recent studies by members of the IDSA have found that the majority of the recommendations in the IDSA guidelines are based more on "expert opinion" than on scientific evidence (Khan et al. 2010; Lee et al. 2011; Johnson & Stricker 2010a).
- Forty percent of the studies cited are written by the authors of the guidelines, who ignore other studies that don't support their viewpoint (Johnson & Stricker 2010a).

Why We Want the IDSA Guidelines Removed From the National Guidelines Clearinghouse

The NGC's own rules require that guidelines be updated every five years in order to remain listed. This has not happened with the IDSA's Lyme guidelines, which were published in 2006 and have not been updated. The IDSA guidelines are out of date, missing important scientific studies that have been subsequently published.

Examples of outdated assertions that hurt Lyme patients:

- IDSA guidelines claim that a) persistence of the Lyme spirochete after treatment is "not plausible," b) antibiotic treatment is ineffective for chronic Lyme, and c) single-dose antibiotic is effective to prevent Lyme (Wormser et al. 2006). All of these assertions have been discredited in subsequent monkey and mouse model trials.
    - Subsequent monkey and mouse studies have found persistence of Lyme spirochetes after treatment, even after 90 days of treatment (Embers et al. 2012).
    - The monkey trial found that antibiotics were effective and cleared spirochetes 25 percent of the time when treated for 90 days.
    - A mouse study demonstrated failure of single-dose preventive antibiotics.
- IDSA guidelines rely heavily on a single human trial conducted by one of the guidelines authors (Klempner 2004), which has subsequently been found to be statistically flawed (DeLong et al. 2012).
- IDSA's own guideline review panel recommended over 25 modifications to the guidelines, which have not been incorporated into the guidelines (IDSA 2010).

- In 2008, the IDSA itself adopted a rigorous evidence assessment process, which has not been applied to the Lyme guidelines (IDSA 2011).

On March 9, 2015, the IDSA announced that it will be updating its Lyme disease guidelines. As the first stage of this process, it announced its formation of a review panel and opened a period of public comment. LymeDisease.org and the national Lyme Disease Association filed comments on behalf of 67 patient groups across the nation. Also during the comment period, LymeDisease.org launched a nationwide survey to solicit views from Lyme patients. It drew more than 6,000 responses in a month. We included findings from that survey in the comments we filed.

IDSA'S Guidelines Process is Troubling

We are deeply troubled by many aspects of the IDSA's guidelines process. The IDSA says it will comply with the Institute of Medicine's standards for creating trustworthy guidelines. Yet, it appears the IDSA is already violating the Institute of Medicine's (IOM) recommendations.

- **The IOM says the panel should include representatives of key affected groups.** But, this panel includes *no* Lyme patients, and *no* physicians who treat them. It also leaves out researchers who don't follow the IDSA's lead regarding Lyme disease. The panel instead includes many IDSA researchers who have consistently excluded patients, opposed their viewpoints, and at times publicly belittled them.
- **The IOM says there should be two patient representatives on the panel, to bring the patient perspective.** Rather than selecting anyone who represents the interests

of the Lyme community, the IDSA chose a "consumer representative" with no knowledge of or experience with Lyme disease. How will that person help the panel understand the views and struggles of Lyme patients? We agree with the IOM that there should be *two* panelists representing Lyme patients. Both of them should have personal experience with Lyme disease and be knowledgeable about related issues. Both should be respected within the Lyme community as capable representatives of patient interests.

- **The IOM also requires that patient preferences and important patient subgroups be considered by the panel.** The IDSA process makes this unlikely to happen. We will send the panelists a summary of "patient perspectives" from our survey. But that is no substitute for effective patient representation.

Sponsoring Organizations Aren't Independent

The IDSA guidelines process is sponsored by three organizations: the IDSA, the American Academy of Neurology, and the American College of Rheumatology. This gives the impression of a broad base of support from independent organizations. Alas, these organizations are hardly independent. As we stated in our comments:

All were implicated by an antitrust investigation by the Connecticut Attorney General in connection with the development of the 2006 IDSA Lyme guidelines. Key members from all three organizations who sat on the panel of the 2006 IDSA Lyme guidelines as well as two of the organizations, the AAN and IDSA, were subject to the investigation by the Attorney General.

The bottom line is that each of these organizations has an interest in supporting a guideline development process that vindicates them and their members from the damage to their reputations incurred in the anti-trust investigation in connection with the development of the IDSA 2006 Lyme guidelines. Developing guidelines that confirm the recommendations in their 2006 Lyme guidelines would accomplish this goal.

Distortion of Process to Conform to Specific Opinions and Biases of Key Panel Members

The panel is supposed to take a systematic, impartial and rigorous look at scientific evidence related to Lyme diagnosis and treatment. Yet that doesn't seem to be the IDSA approach. The 2006 panel ignored studies that didn't support its pre-drawn conclusions. And 40 percent of its citations were to research studies authored by members of the panel.

The new panel seems poised to go down the same inappropriate road. Before it even starts deliberating, key members appear to be trying to "front load" the evidence. How are they doing this? By rushing to publication a number of biased journal articles, which they can then cite as "evidence" backing their position.

This is stacking the deck. It's making sure you have your biased research on the top of the pile, then reviewing it with your own eyes and finding it top rate. Panel members should not be in a position to review and promote their own work while excluding work of their peers. That is not an unbiased review. It makes a mockery of the scientific process.

We Conclude With the Following Recommendations:

The current plan fails to provide the type of process integrity essential to creating trustworthy guidelines. We believe that the plan to should be revised to achieve the following goals.

1.   The IDSA/AAN/ACR panels should be balanced, and represent scientists and physicians from both opposing Lyme paradigms.

2.   Robust patient representation (two or more) is important and should not be token. Patients should be empowered and prepared patients who represent the population affected by Lyme disease.

3.   Consensus should not be obtained by excluding people who disagree.

4.   Controversies and disagreement should be acknowledged. Minority viewpoints should be published with the guidelines.

5.   A public docket of all comments should be maintained and be publicly posted on the IDSA website.

6.   The IDSA/AAN/ACR guidelines should be reconciled with the guidelines of ILADS.

7.   All value judgments by the panel, particularly those pertaining to the patient's role in risk/benefit assessment, should be carefully delineated together with the basis for such judgment.

8.   Panel members should not be selecting or reviewing work of their own or their fellow panel members to avoid abusive self-citation that perpetuates their own biased viewpoint in a highly contested area of medicine.

9.   Panel members with conflicts of interests, including those related to diagnostic testing, should be eliminated from the panel.

10. Panel members who were subject to investigation by the Connecticut Attorney General for antitrust violations in

connection with the 2006 IDSA Lyme disease guidelines development process or the copycat guidelines (e.g. those of the AAN) highlighted in that investigation should also be eliminated from the panel.

11. Guidelines should undergo rigorous external peer review by all interested parties. Responses to comments should be made public.

(To stay current on news about the IDSA guidelines process, follow updates on the LymeDisease.org website.)

Acknowledgements

It would be difficult to enumerate everyone who has helped teach us about this complex subject. We have both learned much from our involvement with LymeDisease.org, the Lyme Disease Association, and the International Lyme and Associated Diseases Society. These groups are made up of people who care deeply about helping those with tick-borne illnesses, and we have found them most willing to share their knowledge with us.

We are inspired by the courage of pioneering doctors Joseph Burrascano, Richard Horowitz, Charles Ray Jones and Kenneth Liegner, who faced professional challenges from the mainstream medical community for their treatment of Lyme disease and did not give in. We appreciate the researchers who continue to bring forth important scientific discoveries about tick-borne illness—Nick Harris, PhD, Alan MacDonald, MD, Eva Sapi, PhD, and others.

We are indebted to the following individuals who provided specific input to this book, either in person or through their writings: Drs. Richard Horowitz, Elizabeth Maloney, Charles Ray Jones, Ann Corson, Robert Bransfield, Kenneth Liegner, as well as Nicola McFadzean, ND, Phyllis Mervine, Patricia Smith, Lorraine Johnson, Shari Brisson, Toni Bernhard, Jennifer Crystal, Melissa Bell, Lisa Kilion and Sophia Webster. Further assistance came from Judith Leventhal, PhD, Sheila Statlender, PhD, Leslie Abrons, LCSW, Education Advocate Patricia Exman, Jack Brennan, Robin Klevansky, Mary Bourguignon, Joanne Ferrante, Alice Renna, and Eli Cohen. Archie Brodsky and Vicki Rowland offered valuable advice regarding writing and publishing. And thanks to EditPros LLC of Davis, California, for publication services.

We also want to recognize the Lyme-related investigative reporting of Mary Beth Pfeiffer of the *Poughkeepsie Journal*. Her insightful and well-informed articles continue to shine a spotlight on the serious public health issues raised by Lyme disease.

Sandy:

I learned much about boundaries, respect, patience and restraint from my friend and mentor of more than 30 years, Jack Brennan, and the core of my work and writing has been informed by our discussions and work together. I am grateful to my co-author, Dorothy Leland, and for the respectful collaboration we created that brought about this book. I am thankful for family and friends who stood by me as I faced my personal struggles with tick-borne disease, especially my husband, Lenny, my son and daughter, Art and Bobbi, and my brother and sister-in-law, Simon and Lorraine. Life has brought me many blessings, and some have come from my struggles with Lyme.

Dorothy:

Thanks to my co-author, Sandy Berenbaum, for the warm working relationship we developed during the writing of this book and other projects, and my deep appreciation to Dr. Steven Harris, William Amalu, DC, Claire Riendeau, ND, and Valerie Frankel, LMFC. Members of the Sacramento Lyme Disease Support Group have taught me much about steadfastness and perseverance over the past seven years. I especially admire how willing they are to help each other by sharing knowledge and words of encouragement. I'm grateful to friends and relatives who helped my family through the hard times. I first learned about how families can survive Lyme disease by being part of one that did, with daughter Rachel, son Jeremy, and husband Bob. My heart overflows with love for them.

Index

About the Authors

Sandra Berenbaum, LCSW, BCD, has a psychotherapy practice that focuses exclusively on Lyme disease patients and their families. In private practice for more than 25 years, Berenbaum is also Children's and Mental Health Editor of *The Lyme Times*, is an advisor to Lyme Connection, and is affiliated with the Lyme Disease Association.

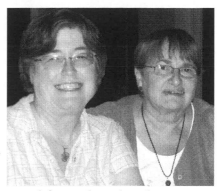

From left, Dorothy and Sandy

She is a member of the International Lyme and Associated Diseases Society, the Council of Parent Attorneys and Advocates, and the National Association of Social Workers. Her presentations at both national and regional conferences have helped educate practitioners about how to work with patients who have Lyme disease. Her website is www.lymefamilies.com. She lives in Connecticut.

Dorothy Kupcha Leland is vice-president of LymeDisease.org, a national patient advocacy group. She has organized patient conferences, testified before the California State Legislature and the state health department, and written Lyme-related articles for a variety of publications. Co-founder of a Lyme support group in Sacramento, California, she also gives tick bite prevention talks. Her blog, *Touched by Lyme*, explores the personal side of Lyme disease and how it affects individuals and families. Follow her on Twitter @dorothyleland. She lives in Northern California.

Our website:
www.lymeliteratepress.com

Follow us on Facebook:
www.facebook.com/WhenYourChildHasLyme

For bulk orders of this book, contact:
info@lymeliteratepress.com

Made in the USA
Columbia, SC
27 March 2018